Lecture Notes in Computer Science 7012

Commenced Publication in 1973
Founding and Former Series Editors:
Gerhard Goos, Juris Hartmanis, and Jan van Leeuwen

Tianming Liu   Dinggang Shen
Luis Ibanez Xiaodong Tao (Eds.)

Multimodal Brain Image Analysis

First International Workshop, MBIA 2011
Held in Conjunction with MICCAI 2011
Toronto, Canada, September 18, 2011
Proceedings

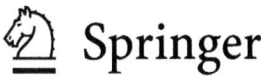 Springer

Volume Editors

Tianming Liu
The University of Georgia
Department of Computer Science and Bioimaging Research Center
Boyd GSRC 422, Athens, GA 30602, USA
E-mail: tliu@cs.uga.edu

Dinggang Shen
University of North Carolina, School of Medicine
Department of Radiology and Biomedical Research Imaging Center
130 Mason Farm Road, Chapel Hill, NC 27599, USA
E-mail: dgshen@med.unc.edu

Luis Ibanez
Kitware Inc., 28 Corporate Drive, Clifton Park, NY 12065, USA
E-mail: luis.ibanez@kitware.com

Xiaodong Tao
General Electric Global Research Center
1 Research Circle, Niskayuna, NY 12309, USA
E-mail: taox@research.ge.com

ISSN 0302-9743   e-ISSN 1611-3349
ISBN 978-3-642-24445-2   ISBN 978-3-642-24446-9 (eBook)
DOI 10.1007/978-3-642-24446-9
Springer Heidelberg Dordrecht London New York

Library of Congress Control Number: 2011936964

CR Subject Classification (1998): I.4, I.5, H.3, I.3.5-8, I.2.10, J.3

LNCS Sublibrary: SL 6 – Image Processing, Computer Vision, Pattern Recognition,
and Graphics

Typesetting: Camera-ready by author, data conversion by Scientific Publishing Services, Chennai, India

Printed on acid-free paper

Springer is part of Springer Science+Business Media (www.springer.com)

Preface

In conjunction with the 14th International Conference on Medical Image Computing and Computer Assisted Intervention (MICCAI), the first international workshop on Multimodal Brain Image Analysis (MBIA) 2011 was held at the Westin Harbour Castle, Toronto, Canada on September 18, 2011.

Noninvasive multimodal brain imaging techniques including structural MRI, diffusion tensor imaging (DTI), perfusion MRI, functional MRI (fMRI), EEG, MEG, PET, SPECT, and CT are playing increasingly important roles in elucidating structural and functional properties in normal and diseased brains. It is widely believed that multiple imaging modalities provide complementary and essential information to understand the brain. Meanwhile, significant challenges arise in processing, fusing, analyzing, and visualizing multimodal brain images due to wide ranges of imaging resolutions, spatial-temporal dynamics, and underlying physical and biological principles.

The objective of this MBIA workshop is to facilitate advancements in the multimodal brain image analysis field, in terms of analysis methodologies, algorithms, software systems, validation approaches, benchmark datasets, neuroscience, and clinical applications. We hope that MBIA workshop can become a forum for researchers in this field to exchange ideas, data, and software, in order to speed up the pace of innovation in applying multimodal brain imaging techniques to testing hypotheses and to data-driven discovery brain science. The objectives of this MBIA workshop include: 1) Bring together researchers in brain imaging, image analysis, neuroscience, and clinical application communities to share ideas, algorithms, data and code, and promote research results achieved in this field to neuroscience and clinical applications; 2) Stimulate thoughts and exploration in new application scenarios, interactions with other related fields, and novel paradigms of multimodal image analysis.

The MBIA 2011 workshop received 24 submissions including 6 invited papers. Each of these papers were peer-reviewed by at least two (typically three) reviewers in the program committee which was composed of 23 experts in the field. Based on the reviewers' recommendations and scores, 15 papers were accepted as oral presentations and 4 papers were accepted as poster presentations. All of the accepted papers were included in the Springer LNCS volume 7012. We would like to express our thanks to all contributing authors.

Finally, we would like to thank the program committee for their contributions in selecting high-quality papers from the submissions and in providing suggestions and critiques that have helped improve the submitted manuscripts.

August 2011

Tianming Liu
Dinggang Shen
Luis Ibanez
Xiaodong Tao

Organization

Program Committee

John Ashburner	UCL, UK
Christian Barillot	IRISA Rennes, France
Vince Calhoun	University of New Mexico, USA
Gary Christensen	University of Iowa, USA
Christos Davatzikos	UPenn, USA
Rachid Deriche	INRIA, France
Atam Dhawan	New Jersey Institute of Technology, USA
James Gee	UPenn, USA
Xiujuan Geng	UNC-Chapel Hill, USA
Guido Gerig	University of Utah, USA
Lei Guo	Northwestern Polytechnic University, China
Bin He	University of Minnesota, USA
Dewen Hu	National University of Defense Technology, China
Xiaoping Hu	Emory University, USA
Tianzi Jiang	Chinese Academy of Science, China
Simon K Warfield	Harvard Medical School and Boston Children's Hospital, USA
Jerry Prince	Johns Hopkins University, USA
Daniel Rueckert	Imperial College London, UK
Li Shen	Indiana University School of Medicine, USA
Feng Shi	UNC-Chapel Hill, USA
Paul Thompson	UCLA, USA
Carl-Fredrik Westin	Harvard Medical School, USA
Guorong Wu	UNC-Chapel Hill, USA
Pew-Thian Yap	UNC-Chapel Hill, USA
Gary Zhang	UCL, UK

Table of Contents

Accounting for Random Regressors: A Unified Approach to Multi-modality Imaging

Xue Yang[1], Carolyn B. Lauzon[1], Ciprian Crainiceanu[2],
Brian Caffo[2], Susan M. Resnick[3], and Bennett A. Landman[1]

[1] Electrical Engineering, Vanderbilt University, Nasvhille TN, 37235 USA
[2] Department of Biostatistics, Johns Hopkins University, Baltimore MD, 21205 USA
[3] National Institute on Aging, National Institutes of Health, Baltimore MD, 21224
{Xue.Yang,Carolyn.Lauzon,Bennett.Landman}@vanderbilt.edu,
{ccrainic,bcaffo}@jhsph.edu,
{resnicks}@grc.nia.nih.gov

Abstract. Massively univariate regression and inference in the form of statistical parametric mapping have transformed the way in which multi-dimensional imaging data are studied. In functional and structural neuroimaging, the *de facto* standard "design matrix"-based general linear regression model and its multi-level cousins have enabled investigation of the biological basis of the human brain. With modern study designs, it is possible to acquire multiple three-dimensional assessments of the same individuals — e.g., structural, functional and quantitative magnetic resonance imaging alongside functional and ligand binding maps with positron emission tomography. Current statistical methods assume that the regressors are non-random. For more realistic multi-parametric assessment (e.g., voxel-wise modeling), distributional consideration of all observations is appropriate (e.g., Model II regression). Herein, we describe a unified regression and inference approach using the design matrix paradigm which accounts for both random and non-random imaging regressors.

Keywords: Model II regression, Inference, Statistical parametric mapping, Biological parametric mapping, model fitting.

1 Introduction

The strong relationship between structure and biological function holds true from the macroscopic scale of multi-cellular organisms to the nano scale of biomacromolecules. Experience informs the clinical researcher that such structure-function relationships must also exist in the brain and, when discovered and quantified, will be powerful informers for early disease detection, prevention, and our overall understanding of the brain. Brain imaging modalities, such as positron emission tomography (PET) and magnetic resonance imaging (MRI), are primary methods for investigating brain structure and function. Quantification of the structure function relationship using imaging data, however, has been challenging owing to the high-dimensional nature of the data and issues of multiple comparisons.

T. Liu et al. (Eds.): MBIA 2011, LNCS 7012, pp. 1–9, 2011.
© Springer-Verlag Berlin Heidelberg 2011

Statistical Parametric Mapping (SPM) enables exploration of relational hypotheses without *a priori* assumptions of regions of interest (ROIs) where the correlations would occur [1, 2]. SPM was limited to single modality regression with imaging data represented only in the regressand until extensions (e.g., Biological Parametric Mapping, BPM) were developed to enable multi-modality regression, allowing for imaging data to use considered for both regressors and regressand [3, 4]. These multi-modal methods rely on the traditional ordinary least squares approach in which regressors are exactly known (i.e., conditional inference). Although this assumption may be reasonable in SPM, where scalar regressors are likely to have significantly less variance than the regressand imaging data, such an assumption is clearly violated when both regressors and regressand are observations from imaging data. With BPM inference is not inverse consistent; interchanging the regressors and regressand images would yield different estimates of relationships. The inconsistent inverse behavior of BPM is a result of violated mathematical assumptions, not underlying biological truths. A researcher is seeking to uncover the two way structure-function relationship and a mathematical technique that optimizes an inverse consistent mapping rather than a unidirectional mapping would bring estimates closer to modeling these underlying physical truths.

Regression analysis accounting for errors in regressors would greatly improve the credibility of the truth model whilst reasonably considering the randomness of the imaging modality. Statistical methods accounting for random regressors have been developed and are collectively known as Model II regression [5, 6]. Surprisingly, Model II regression has not been generalized for the massively univariate case. To more accurately reflect clinical imaging data, herein we develop a general model that accounts for both random regressors and non-random regressors for use in the context of BPM and multi-modality image regression.

2   Theory

Our aim is to explain the observed intensity from one imaging modality, $\mathbf{y}$, with a set of regressors, $\mathbf{x}$, of which at least one member is observed intensity from another imaging modality. We begin with a typical general linear model (GLM) and reformulate it to explicitly reflect the clinical imaging case of both random and non-random regressors. To begin, GLM is formulated as,

$$\mathbf{y} = \sum_{l=1}^{d} \mathbf{x}^{(l)} \boldsymbol{\beta}^{(l)} + \boldsymbol{\varepsilon} \qquad (1)$$

where d is the total number of regressors, $\boldsymbol{\varepsilon}$ is a parameterization of observational error in $\mathbf{y}$, and $\boldsymbol{\beta}$ is a vector of the fitted coefficients. Let $\boldsymbol{\sigma}_{x^{(l)}}$ and σ_y represent the common variance of each element about its truth in $\mathbf{x}^{(l)}$ and $\mathbf{y}$ respectively. Then the $\mathbf{x}^{(l)}$ can be divided into two disjoint sets, fixed regressors whose values are considered to be exactly known, $\mathbf{x_f}$, s.t. ($\boldsymbol{\sigma}_{x_f} \ll \sigma_y$), and random regressors, $\mathbf{x_r}$, s.t. ($\boldsymbol{\sigma}_{x_r}$ not $\ll \sigma_y$). In BPM, all regressors are treated as fixed regressors. By inclusion of random regressors, that Model-II diverges from BPM. Owing to their larger σ values, the observed $\mathbf{x_r}$ are only therefore noisy estimates of the truth, $\mathbf{x_{r-T}}$. Eq. 1 then becomes,

$$\mathbf{y} = \sum_{j=1}^{q} \mathbf{x}_{rT}^{(j)} \beta_r^{(j)} + \sum_{k=1}^{m} \mathbf{x}_f^{(k)} \beta_f^{(k)} + \boldsymbol{\varepsilon} \tag{2}$$

where q and m represent the total number of random and fixed regressors respectively. The challenge here, that is not present in Model-I, is to estimate $\boldsymbol{\beta}_r$ and $\boldsymbol{\beta}_f$ given that $\mathbf{x}_{rT}$ in Eq. 2 is not observed, but rather the noisy $\mathbf{x}_r$. There are many possible methods for solving for $\boldsymbol{\beta}$, here we choose an approach that follows the ordinary least squares example. We seek a solution for the parameters, $\boldsymbol{\beta}$, that maximize the log-likelihood of the model given the observed data (maximize $\ln P(\mathbf{y}, \mathbf{x}_r | \boldsymbol{\beta}, \Sigma, \mathbf{y}_T, \mathbf{x}_{rT})$).

Let $i = 1, 2, \ldots n$ index the observations in $\mathbf{y}$ and in each of the $\mathbf{x}_r^{(j)}$ (e.g. $n =$ the number of subjects and i indexes the subject number). Let $\mathbf{z}_i$ be a vector representing the i'th set of observational errors in $\mathbf{y}$ and in each $\mathbf{x}_r^{(j)}$. We can assume the errors follow a multivariate normal distribution with mean $\mathbf{0}$ and covariance matrix, Σ [7].

$$\mathbf{z}_i = \begin{bmatrix} \mathbf{y} - \mathbf{y}_T & x_r^{(1)} - x_{rT}^{(1)} & \cdots & x_r^{(q)} - x_{rT}^{(q)} \end{bmatrix} \sim \Phi(\mathbf{0}, \Sigma) \tag{3}$$

Note that the observational errors, $\mathbf{z}$, are errors across subjects and do not condition errors across an image. Given that each $\mathbf{x}_r^{(j)}$ vector is observed from a unique experimental technique, it is reasonable to assume that the columns of $\mathbf{z}_i$ are independent. We further assume that $\mathbf{z}_i$ is independent as each subject is independent. independent. Under these assumptions (normal and i.i.d.), the log-likelihood of the observed data, given the model in Eq. 2 is,

$$\ln P(\mathbf{y}, \mathbf{x}_r | \boldsymbol{\beta}, \Sigma, \mathbf{y}_T, \mathbf{x}_{rT}) = \sum_{i=1}^{n} \ln\left(2\pi^{-n/2}\left(\det(\Sigma)^{-1/2}\right)\right) - \frac{1}{2}\sum_{i=1}^{n}(\mathbf{z}_i \Sigma^{-1} \mathbf{z}_i') \tag{4}$$

Maximizing the log likelihood, Eq. 4, is equivalent to minimizing $s = \sum_{i=1}^{n}(\mathbf{z}_i \Sigma^{-1} \mathbf{z}_i')$. With the assumption of independent observations (independent subjects, i, and independent experiments, $\mathbf{x}_r^{(j)}$, the covariance matrix, Σ, is diagonal with entries $\sigma_y^2 \; \sigma_{x_r^{(1)}}^2 \ldots \sigma_{x_r^{(q)}}^2$. Hence, s can be re-expressed as,

$$s = \sum_{i=1}^{n}\left(\sigma_y^{-2}(y_i - y_{T_i})^2 + \sum_{j=1}^{q}\sigma_{x_r^{(j)}}^{-2}\left(x_{r_i}^{(j)} - x_{rT_i}^{(j)}\right)^2\right) \tag{5}$$

where $x_{r_i}^{(j)}$ represents the ith element of $\mathbf{x}_r^{(j)}$. Eq. 5 is minimized when its partial derivatives w.r.t to each dependent variable is zero. We first solve for $\mathbf{x}_{rT}$ at the minimum of Eq.5 by differentiating s with respect to $x_{rT}^{(j)}$ and setting the result to $\mathbf{0}$ gives q total equations, one for each $\mathbf{x}_r^{(j)}$. With q equations and q unknowns, $x_{rT}^{(j)}$ can be solved in terms of the other parameters. For a given term indexed by h,

$$x_{rT}^{(h)} = \frac{\beta_r^{(h)}\sigma_{x_r^{(h)}}^2\left(y + x_r^{(h)}\beta_r^{(h)} - \sum_{j=1}^{q} x_r^{(j)}\beta_r^{(j)} - \sum_{k=1}^{m} x_k^{(j)}\beta_r^{(j)}\right) + x_r^{(h)}\left(\sum_{j=1}^{q}\left(\beta_r^{(j)}\sigma_{x_r^{(j)}}^2\right) - \beta_r^{(h)}\sigma_{x_r^{(h)}}^2 + \sigma_y^2\right)}{\sigma_y^2 + \sum_{j=1}^{q}\beta_r^{(j)2}\sigma_{x_r^{(j)}}^2} \tag{6}$$

Substituting Eq. 6 for $\mathbf{x}_{rT}^{(j)}$ in Eq. 5, s becomes,

$$s = \frac{1}{\sigma_y^2} \sum_{i=1}^{n} \frac{\left(y_i - \left(\sum_{j=1}^{q} x_{r_i}^{(j)} \beta_r^{(j)} + \sum_{k=1}^{m} x_{f_i}^{(k)} \beta_f^{(k)}\right)\right)^2}{\sigma_y^2 + \sum_{j=1}^{q} \beta_r^{(j)2} \sigma_{x_r^{(j)}}^2} \qquad (7)$$

Eq. 7 is now independent of the unknown x_{rT} and provides an intuitive form as the model error in the numerator is balanced by the individual variances in the denominator and mirrors the more readily available multivariate case with non-random x and the univariate case that accounts for a single random x [8]. Eq. 7 is a function of two unknowns, β and σ. Note that the true σ does not factor into s, only the ratio of variance matters. If these ratios are known, then β is the only unknown; and the β that maximizes Eq. 4 can be solved by taking the partial derivative of s with respect to β and setting the result to 0. The partial derivative equations are nonlinear w.r.t. β, and solving for the closed form solution of β is involved, so we employ numeric optimization methods.

In the Model II approach, the variance ratio needs to be known in order to minimize s by solving β. The restriction arises because the number of unknown parameters is larger than the number of equations [9]. If we add the further assumption that the ratio of the overall variance across subjects is proportional to the ratio of the image noise variance, then we can estimate the model variance ratio by estimating the ratio of image noise for each modality.

Inference on β

The maximum likelihood estimate of β, β_{est}, with a true value β_T, is asymptotically normally distributed as $(\beta_{est} - \beta_T) \sim \Phi(0, nI^{-1})$ where I is the Fisher information matrix $(I_{w,g} = E[-\nabla_{\beta^{(w)}\beta^{(g)}} \ln P_i(y_i, x_{ri}|\beta, \Sigma, y_T, x_{rTi})])$, with $w = 1,2,\ldots q+m$, $g = 1,2,\ldots q+m$, P_i is the probability function for data i. Noting the distribution $y_i - \left(\sum_{j=1}^{q} x_{r_i}^{(j)} \beta_{est,r}^{(j)} + \sum_{k=1}^{m} x_{r_i}^{(k)} \beta_{est,f}^{(k)}\right) \sim N\left(0, \sigma_y^2 + \sum_{j=1}^{q} \beta_{est,r}^{(j)2} \sigma_{x_r^{(j)}}^2\right)$, the Fisher information can be estimated from prior ratio and dataset. Allowing c to represent the contrast vector and $\beta_T = \beta_{null}$ to be the null hypothesis, then it follows that the test-statistic, $c'(\beta_{est}-\beta_{null}) / \sqrt{c'(n\hat{I})^{-1}c}$ is t-distributed with n-$(q+m)$ degrees of freedom. This is an asymptotic t-test as all estimated parameters and Fisher information are asymptotically valid.

3   Methods and Results

3.1   Single Voxel Simulations with Known True Variance Ratios

Model II regression is implemented using the Nelder–Mead method to find the optimized solution of β. For each of the following 3 scenarios, a simulated voxel with 50 observations (i.e., subjects) was studied using a model with one random regressor, one fixed regressor, and a single constant: $y_T = x_{rT}\beta_r + x_f\beta_f + \beta_1$. In each of 500 Monte Carlo trials: β_T were chosen randomly from the uniform distribution (0-2); errors were added to y_{T_i} and x_{rT_i} from a normal distribution with fixed standard deviations, and the true variance ratio was assumed known. Model II and OLS performance were evaluated with the relative root mean squared error in β ($r\beta_{RMS}$).

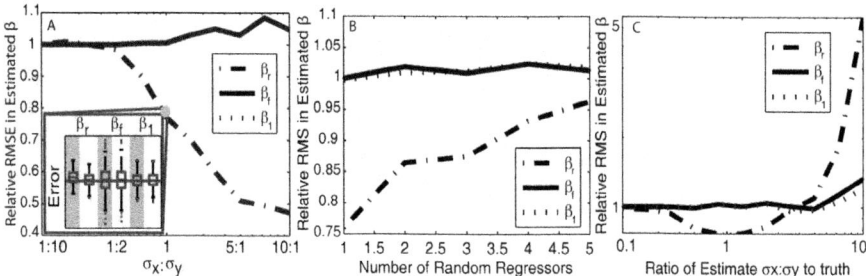

Fig. 1. The relative RMSEs of Model II to OLS for each estimated coefficient (β_r, β_f, β_1) are plotted as a function of the ratio of the true standard deviations, $\sigma_x{:}\sigma_y$ (A), the number of random regressors, $x_r^{(j)}$ (B) and the accuracy of the ratio estimate (C). With increasing $\sigma_x{:}\sigma_y$ ratios, model II regression has increased relative accuracy in β_r estimates compared to OLS with increasing $\sigma_x{:}\sigma_y$ ratios. Comparison of the β_f, β_r, and β_1 error distributions formed is shown explicitly in the inlay for the point $\sigma_x/\sigma_y =1$ in (A). The gray column shows the OLS error and the white column shows the Model II error, the horizontal line is where the error is zero. In (C), for one unit σ_y, the estimated ratio μ_x was allowed to deviate from the ideal case, $\mu_x/\sigma_x = 1$. The common point shared in (A, B, C) is located in (B) at 'Number of Random Regressors' = 1, and (C) at 'Ratio of Estimate to Truth' = 1.

(A) **Model II vs OLS response to $\sigma_x : \sigma_y$ ratios (Figure 1A).** Simulations were performed varying $\sigma_x{:}\sigma_y$. Model II regression performs equally well as OLS with small $\sigma_x{:}\sigma_y$, but becomes advantageous as more relative error is introduced into $\mathbf{x_r}$ observations. The improvement is observed specifically on β_r, whereas the constants not associated with random regressors, β_1 and β_f, remain with equal accuracy in estimation between the two models.

(B) **Model II vs OLS response to number of random x regressors (Figure 1B).** The above model was altered by including up to 4 additional random regressors with randomized coefficients. Model II has smaller errors in the β_r estimates than OLS, however Model II becomes less advantageous with increases in the number of random x regressors. Note, the number of observations was not increased to compensate for the increased model complexity so less data per regressor is available with more regressors.

(C) **Model II sensitivity to the estimated ratio (Figure 1C).** To assess the response of Model II to estimated ratios that deviate from the truth, the assumed true ratio of variance was altered between $1/10^{th}$ and 10 times its true value. Under the cases simulated here, Model II is insensitive to the ratio estimate for the range (0.5-2) and relatively insensitive over the range (.1-3). At extremely incorrect ratio values, the β_r estimate rapidly looses accuracy. Based on this analysis we can apply Model II regression using estimated error ratio, with reasonable confidence in the methods' tolerance to mis-estimation of variance ratios.

3.2 Volumetric Imaging Simulation

Model II regression is incorporated as a regression method choice in the BPM toolbox for the SPM software using Matlab (Mathworks, Natick, MA). We simulated images

6   X. Yang et al.

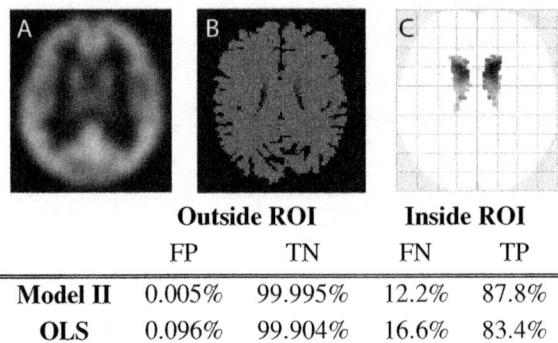

| | Outside ROI | | Inside ROI | |
	FP	TN	FN	TP
Model II	0.005%	99.995%	12.2%	87.8%
OLS	0.096%	99.904%	16.6%	83.4%

Fig. 2. (A) is one regressor image, (B) is one regressand image in Model II BPM simulation. (C) is one dimension of the glass brain which is the projected statistical significance. The glass brain is shown according to uncorrected p-value p<0.001 and 5 voxels extent threshold to exclude noise. The table is calculated with p<0.001.

of two modalities and regressed one modality on the other modality. The true regressor images are simulated from smoothed gray matter density images of 20 participants in the normal aging study of the BLSA neuroimaging project consisting of 79*95*69 voxels with 0.94*0.94*1.5 mm resolution [10]. The observed regressor images are simulated by adding zero mean Gaussian noise. The true regressand image intensity is "1.5*true regressor images – constant" inside the caudate region and equals a different constant everywhere else inside the brain mask. The observed regressand images were generated by adding zero mean Gaussian noise to the true regressand images. The standard deviation of the noise is selected to make SNR=15. (SNR is defined as the mean signal divided by the standard deviation of noise). The observed regressor images and observed regressand images are used for simulation and the ratio of noise standard deviation is used as the ratio of observation error in Model II regression.

Fig. 2 presents the results for 20 simulated subject brains, each represented by a pairs of images. The statistical significance map is shown according to uncorrected p-value with p<0.001 and 5 voxels extent threshold to exclude noise. Type I error and type II error are calculated at uncorrected p-value<0.001 inside (for true-positive, TP, and false-negative, FN) and outside a caudate mask (for false-positive, FP, and true-negative, TN). In this simple model, both OLS and Model II regression control type I error as expected. Meanwhile, Model II regression improves true positive rate as compared to OLS regression.

3.3 Empirical Demonstration of Model II Regression

Image-on-image regression offers a direct opportunity to study associations between differing spatially located factors. As an illustrative example, consider potential correlations between GM tissue density (a structural measure) and PET signal (a measure of functional activity). A first model would associate tissue presence with greater functional signal. An analysis of modulating factors for this relationship (such as disease condition, intervention, or task) could reveal anatomical correlates of functional reorganization and shed light on the applicability of the structural-functional hypothesis.

Following this approach, we perform regression analysis of the relationship between anatomical MRI gray matter images (GM, as classified by SPM5) and functional PET images. PET and GM data were collected on a total of $n = 46$ observations (23 subjects imaged twice). Regression was performed in both directions in order to quantify both structure→function and function→structure relationships. The regression model used 1 random regressor and a single constant. For the Model II ratio, noise ratio is estimated following the method in [11]. The raw data and the resulting regression lines for a single voxel comparison are displayed. Fi.e 3 shows that Model II is symmetric, i.e., the mapping PET→GM is the inverse of the mapping GM → PET. The corresponding estimated variances for Model II are also smaller than the corresponding estimated variances in OLS forward regression and OLS inverse regression.

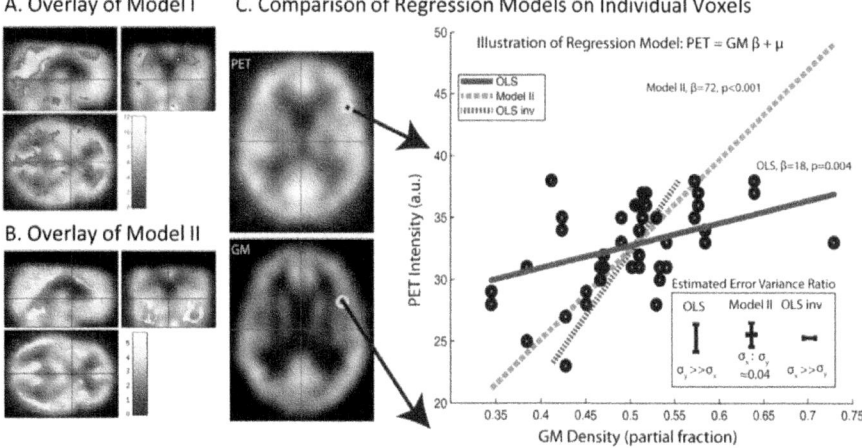

Fig. 3. Model II and Model I (OLS) multi-modality regression analysis. Model I (A) and Model II (B) lead to distinct patterns of significant differences (p<0.001, uncorrected) when applied to identical empirical datasets and association models. Inspection of single voxel: PET vs Grey Matter MRI (GM) illustrates the reasons for the different findings (C). The GLM model used for the forward mapping is $\mathbf{y} = \mathbf{x_r}\beta_r + \beta_1$, where $\mathbf{y}$ represents PET image intensity and $\mathbf{x_r}$ represents GM normalized image intensity. On the left-hand side of (C), example images of PET and GM are shown, along with the location of the single example voxel whose regression analysis is displayed in the right-hand plot. The individual data points (blue circles) were fit using OLS (red lines) and Model II regression (green dashed line). The inverse mapping for OLS (red dash) is unique from the forward mapping (red full). The Model II mapping was found to be reversible and can be represented by the same line. Resulting error bars and corresponding $\sigma_x{:}\sigma_y$ value estimates are compared between OLS and Model II in the lower right-hand insert.

4 Discussion

Properly accounting for error is essential for valid parameter estimation and statistical inference. Herein, we have demonstrated that a full consideration of observation variability is feasible within the confines of a design matrix paradigm. Furthermore, we can readily consider simultaneous treatment of parameters with measurement error ($\mathbf{x}_r$) alongside traditionally defined fixed parameters ($\mathbf{x}_f$). Our formulation of "random observations" remains within the context of a "fixed effects" model as the $\boldsymbol{\beta}_r$ $\boldsymbol{\beta}_r$ are deterministic parameters, as opposed to the classic "random effects" model where parameters are stochastic. These two approaches are complementary and could be combined for an appropriate experimental framework. Extension of the Model II concepts to time series, hierarchical and complex model designs would be a fascinating area for continuing research.

We have observed substantial improvements in model fit and increased statistical power using Model II regression as opposed to OLS (Fig. 1A). While robust to model complexity (Fig. 1B) and prior estimation of observation variability (Fig. 1C), the improvements were not universal. When the OLS is appropriate (i.e., $\sigma_x \ll \sigma_y$), there was a slight increase in observed error (Fig. 1A); however, as the relative variance in $\mathbf{x}$ increased, the OLS assumption of fixed regressors becomes increasingly violated and notable bias and increased variance could be observed in the OLS estimates. Examination of the inlays in Fig. 1 reveals a slight increase in error for the fixed parameters, β_f and β_1, but a lack of appreciable bias.

The generalized Model II regression model can be used to analyze any complicated relationship by applying Taylor series and expand design matrix. Our presentation of Model II regression is inverse consistent, provides a logical framework for exploring relationships in multi-modal image analysis, and can help model relative uncertainty in imaging methods. Other error models may be more appropriate for specific imaging modalities and warrant further consideration.

Our presentation of the empirical analysis is preliminary and ongoing as is highlighted by the single voxel presentation. Interpreting the ratio of model variances is subject of active consideration as must consider the potential impact of both the imaging variability and model fit error in multiple dimensions. As discussed, we currently approximate this combined quantity as proportional to the imaging variability alone. Relaxing this assumption would greatly aid in generalization of this approached. These methods are available in open source as plug-ins for the SPM package.

Acknowledgements. This project was supported by NIH N01-AG-4-0012. *This work described herein has not been submitted elsewhere for publication.*

References

1. Friston, K., Frith, C., Liddle, P., Dolan, R., Lammertsma, A., Frackowiak, R.: The relationship between global and local changes in PET scans. Journal of cerebral blood flow and metabolism: official Journal of the International Society of Cerebral Blood Flow and Metabolism 10, 458 (1990)

2. Friston, K., Frith, C., Liddle, P., Frackowiak, R.: Comparing functional (PET) images: the assessment of significant change. Journal of cerebral blood flow and metabolism: official Journal of the International Society of Cerebral Blood Flow and Metabolism 11, 690 (1991)
3. Casanova, R., Srikanth, R., Baer, A., Laurienti, P., Burdette, J., Hayasaka, S., Flowers, L., Wood, F., Maldjian, J.: Biological parametric mapping: a statistical toolbox for multimodality brain image analysis. NeuroImage 34, 137–143 (2007)
4. Oakes, T.R., Fox, A.S., Johnstone, T., Chung, M.K., Kalin, N., Davidson, R.J.: Integrating VBM into the General Linear Model with voxelwise anatomical covariates. Neuroimage 34, 500–508 (2007)
5. York, D.: Least-squares fitting of a straight line. Canadian Jour. Physics 44, 1079–1086 (1966)
6. Ludbrook, J.: Linear regression analysis for comparing two measurers or methods of measurement: But which regression? Clinical and Experimental Pharmacology and Physiology 37, 692–699 (2010)
7. Friston, K., Holmes, A., Worsley, K., Poline, J., Frith, C., Frackowiak, R.: Statistical parametric maps in functional imaging: a general linear approach. Human Brain Mapping 2, 189–210 (1994)
8. Press, W.: Numerical recipes: the art of scientific computing. Cambridge Univ. Pr., Cambridge (2007)
9. Carroll, R., Ruppert, D.: The Use and Misuse of Orthogonal Regression in Linear Errors-in-Variables Models. The American Statistician 50 (1996)
10. Resnick, S.M., Goldszal, A.F., Davatzikos, C., Golski, S., Kraut, M.A., Metter, E.J., Bryan, R.N., Zonderman, A.B.: One-year age changes in MRI brain volumes in older adults. Cerebral Cortex 10, 464 (2000)
11. Rajan, J., Poot, D., Juntu, J., Sijbers, J.: Noise measurement from magnitude MRI using local estimates of variance and skewness. Physics in Medicine and Biology 55, N441 (2010)

Joint T1 and Brain Fiber Diffeomorphic Registration Using the Demons

Viviana Siless[1,2], Pamela Guevara[2,3], Xavier Pennec[4], and Pierre Fillard[1,2]

[1] Parietal Team, INRIA Saclay-Île-de-France, Saclay, France
viviana.siless@inria.fr
http://parietal.saclay.inria.fr
[2] CEA, DSV, I²BM, Neurospin bât 145, 91191 Gif-Sur-Yvette, France
[3] University of Concepción, Concepción, Chile
[4] Asclepios Team, INRIA Sophia Antipolis Méditerraneé, Sophia Antipolis, France

Abstract. Non-linear image registration is one of the most challenging task in medical image analysis. In this work, we propose an extension of the well-established diffeomorphic Demons registration algorithm to take into account geometric constraints. Combining the deformation field induced by the image and the geometry, we define a mathematically sound framework to jointly register images and geometric descriptors such as fibers or sulcal lines. We demonstrate this framework by registering simultaneously T_1 images and 50 fiber bundles consistently extracted in 12 subjects. Results show the improvement of fibers alignment while maintaining, and sometimes improving image registration. Further comparisons with non-linear T_1 and tensor registration demonstrate the superiority of the Geometric Demons over their purely iconic counterparts.

Keywords: Registration, neural fibers, diffeomorphism, Demons Algorithm, intensity-base registration, tensor-base registration.

1 Introduction

Image registration is undoubtedly one of the most active area of research in medical imaging. Within inter-individual comparison, registration should align images as well as cortical and internal structures such as sulcal lines and fibers.

Non-linear registration algorithms can be categorized into three types: iconic, geometric and hybrid. Iconic, or image-based registration [1,2,3] consists in finding a voxel-wise mapping between a source and a target image. Schematically, iconic registration is mainly driven by the image contours (e.g., boundaries between white and grey matter). This approach suffers from the aperture problem: without prior knowledge, it is difficult to choose between two structures with similar contrast in the target image. Similarly, brain white matter, while being composed of neural fibers connecting cortical areas together, appears uniformly white in T_1 images, giving no relevant information to the iconic registratrion. Diffusion Tensor Imaging (DTI) can be used to reveal the microscopic structure of the white matter. Tensor-based registration was recently proposed to improve

T. Liu et al. (Eds.): MBIA 2011, LNCS 7012, pp. 10–18, 2011.

white matter alignment [4,5]. However, misregistration may persist in regions where the tensor field appears uniform, as shown in [6].

Geometric registration specifically targets the alignment of Structures of Interest (SOI), such as in [7] for cortical surfaces, or [6] for fiber bundles. While those clearly improve SOI registration, they are in general not suitable for inferring a volumetric mapping between two subjects and cannot be used for comparing other structures than those used specifically during registration.

Hybrid techniques propose to jointly consider SOI and images during registration. For instance, [8,9] used the mathematical framework of the *currents* to simultaneously register images and geometric descriptors, while [10] proposed a Markovian solution to the same problem.

In this work, we propose to extend a well-established and efficient registration algorithm: the Demons. First introduced by Thirion et al. [1], and further extended by Vercauteren et al. [11] in a diffeomorphic version, the Demons have been widely used in the community for their efficiency and accuracy.

The rest of the paper is organised as follows. First, we propose a mathematically sound extension of the Demons, the Geometric Demons (GD), taking into account geometric constraints. Second, we evaluate the Geometric Demons with fiber constraints on a dataset of 12 subjects and compare them with their scalar and tensor versions [5], before concluding.

2   The Geometric Demons

2.1   The Diffeomorphic Demons

Image registration looks for a displacement field s between a fixed F and moving M image, that maps as accurately as possible corresponding structures in both images. Finding s is often treated as an optimization problem whose solution is defined by the minimum of the following energy: $E(s) = \frac{1}{\sigma_i^2}\mathrm{Sim}_I(F, M \circ s) + \frac{1}{\sigma_T^2}\mathrm{Reg}(s)$, where Sim_I is a similarity measure between images and Reg a regularization term. The amount of regularization is controlled with σ_T while σ_i accounts for the image noise. In this work, the image similarity is defined as the sum of square differences (SSD): $\mathrm{Sim}_I(F, M) = \|F - M\|^2$, $\|.\|$ being the L_2 norm. The regularization is chosen to be the harmonic energy: $\mathrm{Reg}(s) = \|\nabla s\|^2$.

In practice, this minimization is often intractable. To overcome this, Thirion et al. [1] introduced an auxiliary variable, the correspondence field c, to account for uncertainty of the displacement field. In other words, c is an exact realization of point-to-point correspondences between images while s allows for some errors. This leads to the following energy functional:

$$E(c, s) = \frac{1}{\sigma_i^2}\mathrm{Sim}(F, M \circ c) + \frac{1}{\sigma_x^2}\mathrm{dist}(s, c)^2 + \frac{1}{\sigma_T^2}\mathrm{Reg}(s), \qquad (1)$$

The term $\mathrm{dist}(s, c)^2$ imposes the displacement field s to be close to the correspondence field c. σ_x weights the spatial uncertainty on the deformation.

The energy minimization is performed by alternating minimization w.r.t. c and s. In [11], small deformations parametrized by a dense displacement field u are used: c is given by s composed with the exponential map of u (in the Lie group sense): $c \leftarrow s \circ \exp(u)$. Using the exponential map ensures the result to be diffeomorphic. The algorithm consists thus in the following steps:

1. Given s, find the optimal update field u minimizing Eq. 1.
2. Let $c \leftarrow s \circ \exp(u)$
3. Minimize Eq. 1 by convolving c with a Gaussian kernel K_{diff}: $s \leftarrow K_{diff} \star c$
4. Iterate until convergence.

Implementation details for each step is given in [11]. In the next section, we show how to adapt the Demons framework to include geometric constraints.

2.2   Adding Geometric Constraints to the Demons

To add geometric constraints in the Demons framework, c should ideally carry information from both image and geometry. Let us denote by $\mathcal{G}^F$ (resp. $\mathcal{G}^M$) the fixed (resp. moving) geometric descriptors. We propose the following formulation:

$$E(c,s) = \frac{1}{\sigma_i^2} \left[\mathrm{Sim}_I(F, M \circ c) + \mathrm{Sim}_G(c \star \mathcal{G}^F, \mathcal{G}^M) \right] +$$
$$\frac{1}{\sigma_x^2} \mathrm{dist}(s,c)^2 + \frac{1}{\sigma_T} \mathrm{Reg}(s), \qquad (2)$$

where Sim_I is the image similarity measure, Sim_G the geometry similarity measure, and $c \star \mathcal{G}^F$ denotes the action of c on the geometry.

Following [11], we parametrize c by an update field, which in this case will be the additive combination of an image update field u_I and a geometric update field u_G. Ideally, one should use u_G only where geometric information is relevant and use u_I elsewhere. Thus, if we denote by Ω_G the definition domain of u_G (regions where geometric correspondences are present), the definition domain of u_I is $\Omega_I = \Omega - \Omega_G$, of which is equivalent to having non-intersecting domains, the union covers the entire domain Ω: $\Omega_I \cap \Omega_P = \emptyset$, $\Omega_I \cup \Omega_G = \Omega$. Under this assumption, c can be seen as the combination of both update fields: $c = \exp(u_I + u_G)$. We can also say that $c \star \mathcal{G}^F = \exp(u_G) \star \mathcal{G}^F$ and $M \circ c = M \circ \exp(u_I)$.

Furthermore, since u_I and u_G have distinct domains, we can write: $\mathrm{dist}(s,c)^2 = \int_{\Omega_G} \|u_G\|^2 + \int_{\Omega_I} \|u_I\|^2$. Optimizing Eq. 2 w.r.t. to u_I leads to the minimization of $E_I(s, u_I) = \frac{1}{\sigma_i^2} \mathrm{Sim}_I(F, M \circ s \circ \exp(u_I)) + \frac{1}{\sigma_x^2} \int_{\Omega_I} \|u_I\|^2$, which is the same formulation as the diffeomorphic Demons. Optimizing Eq. 2 w.r.t. to u_G leads to minimizing the following energy:

$$E_G(s, u_G) = \frac{1}{\sigma_i^2} \mathrm{Sim}_G(s \circ \exp(u_G) \star \mathcal{G}^F, \mathcal{G}^M) + \frac{1}{\sigma_x^2} \int_{\Omega_G} \|u_G\|^2, \qquad (3)$$

Finally, the Geometric Demons algorithm can be formulated as such:

1. Given s, u_G, compute the update field u_I as for the diffeomorphic Demons
2. Given s, u_I, compute the update field u_G by minimizing Eq. 3

3. Let $c \leftarrow s \circ \exp(u_I + u_G)$
4. Given c, let $s \leftarrow K_{diff} \star c$
5. Iterate until convergence

Steps 1, 3 and 4 are similar to the diffeomorphic Demons. Note that step 4 ensures that the combined correspondence field is smooth. In the following, we detail the computation of u_G in the case of point sets as geometric descriptors.

Calculation of u_G for Point Sets. There are numerous ways to measure similarity between geometrical primitives such as with the Hausdorff distance, the Closest Point distance (CPD), or even more sophisticatedly, with the currents. Our aim is to jointly minimize image and geometric energies within the Demons's framework, thus we focus on the overall algorithm behaviour using a simple metric for now.

Let us consider our geometric descriptors as point sets: $\mathcal{G} = \{x_i\}_{i \in [1,N]}$, being N the number of points. Let us denote by π_i the point index in $\mathcal{G}^M$ closest to point i in $\mathcal{G}^F$. We define the similarity measure between point set with the CPD:

$$\text{Sim}_G(\mathcal{G}^F, \mathcal{G}^M) = \frac{1}{N} \sum_{i=1}^{N} ||x_i^F - x_{\pi_i}^M||_2^2 \tag{4}$$

Let us define the action of the correspondence field c on a point set as: $c \star \mathcal{G} = \{s \circ \exp(u_G)(x_i)\}_{i \in [1,N]} \approx \{s(x_i) + u_G(x_i)\}_{i \in [1,N]}$. Since we are dealing with sets of points, we choose to parametrize the dense update field u_G by a finite set of vectors $u_{G,i}$ using radial basis function interpolation: $u_G(x) = \sum_{i=1}^{N} h(||x - x_i||)\lambda_i$. $h(.)$ is a radial function (we use $h(x) = ||x||$). λ_i are calculated such that $u_G(x_i) = u_{G,i} \forall i$. Let us define the matrix A such that $[A]_{i,j} = h(||x_i - x_j||)$ ($[A]_{i,j}$ denotes the ith row and j^{th} column of A), $\Lambda = [\lambda_1, ..., \lambda_N]$ the vector of λs, $H(x)$ the vector such that $[H(x)]_i = h(||x - x_i||)$ and $U = [u_{G,1}, ..., u_{G,N}]$. We can write: $u_G(x) = H(x)A^{-1}U$. Solving $\nabla E_G(s, u_G) = 0$ w.r.t. u_G narrows down to optimization for the $u_{G,i}, \forall i$. After differentiation, we obtain:

$$u_{G,i} = \frac{x_{\pi_i}^M - s(x_i^F)}{1 + \frac{N\sigma_i^2}{\sigma_x^2}[H(s(x_i^F))A^{-1}]_i}$$

Defining Ω_G for Point sets. Since we want points to influence the deformation near the definition domain, we define the domain as the union of γ−radius balls B centered at each coordinate x_i. We control the influence by varying γ and thus, dilating the domain. We define a binary map $\Omega_G^\gamma = \bigcup_{i=1}^{N} B(x_i, \gamma)$. The domain of the image correspondence field is the complementary of Ω_G^γ: $\Omega_I^\gamma = \Omega \backslash \Omega_G^\gamma$.

3   Joint T_1 MRI and Brain Fiber Registration

We now apply the GD the joint registration of T_1 MRI and brain fibers.

3.1 Data Description

Analysis was performed for 12 subjects of the NMR public database [12]. This database provides high quality T1-weighted images and diffusion data acquired with a GE Healthcare Signa 1.5 Tesla Excite II scanner. The diffusion data presents a high angular resolution (HARDI) based on 200 directions and a b-value of 3000 s/mm2 (voxel size of $1.875 \times 1.875 \times 2$ mm). Distorsion correction and fiber tractography and clustering were performed using the Brainvisa software package (http://brainvisa.info). Using [13], we obtained corresponding fiber bundles between several subjects and a single representative fiber for each bundle. About 100 bundles were consistently identified in all subjects. The 50 longest (25 in each hemisphere) were retained for the experiments. For each subject we apply affine registration from B_0 to T_1 and use the resulting transformation to align budles with T_1 images. Bundles were further simplified into point sets, which allows us to use the methodology presented in Sec. 2.

3.2 Experiments

Two experiments were conducted. First, we performed an exhaustive analysis of the parameter γ of Sec. 2.2 to understand its effect on registration accuracy. Second, we compared the performance between the GD, the Scalar Demons (SD) and the Tensor Demons (TD). For both experiments, 11 subjects were registered onto one, arbitrary chosen as the target. Note that the deformation field obtained is the *resampling* deformation: it goes from target to source. As our deformation field is diffeomorphic we can invert it to display registered fibers onto the target.

Influence of γ. We varied γ from 0 (no fiber influence, which is equivalent to SD) to 3.0. Registration results for three values of γ are shown in Fig. 1. Values of the image and fiber similarity measures for increasing values of γ are reported in Fig. 1 (d) and (e). As expected, when γ increases, fiber matching improves at the expense of image alignment. Indeed, when fibers have a large influence on their neighborhood, image-driven forces are discarded, leading to poor image registration. However, we noticed that a γ value of 1.5 largely improves fiber alignment while keeping a good match between images. Notably, in some cases image matching is improved when using fiber as constraints compared to not using them at all, pointing out the fact that geometry may indeed help image registration to avoid local minima. In the sequel, a γ of 1.5 will be used.

Comparison with Scalar and Tensor Demons. For SD, we registered all 11 T_1 images onto the target and applied the inverted deformation field to the bundles. For TD, we extracted tensors using [14] and registered them onto the target tensor image. Then, inverted deformation fields were applied to each subject's fibers in the DWI space. Finally, the linear transformation calculated between the target B_0 and T_1 images was applied to fibers to carry them to the T_1 space. We evaluated the fiber similarity measure between registered source and target fibers. Results for each method and each subject are reported in Fig. 2.

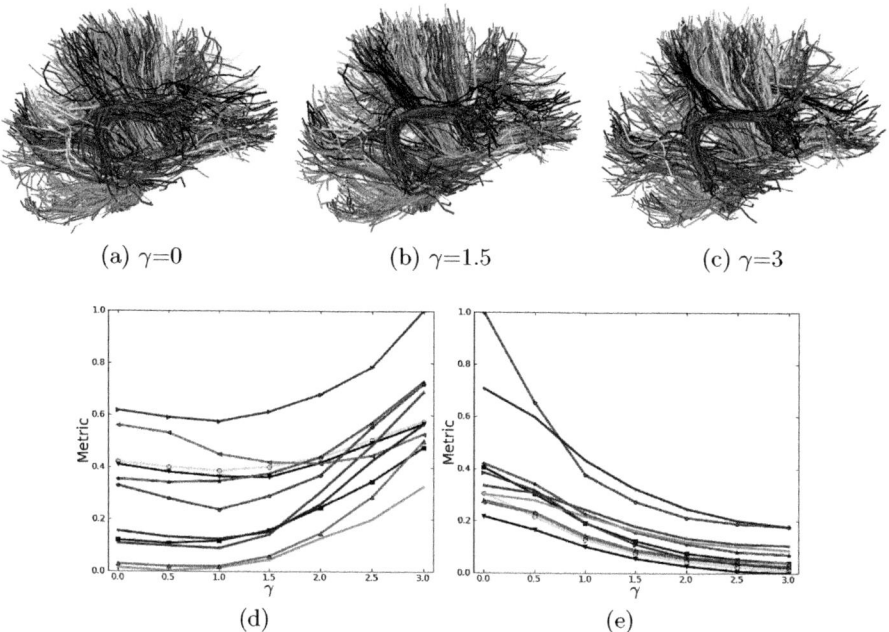

Fig. 1. Influence of γ on the registration accuracy. Top: Fibers of 11 subjects were overlapped after registration with the Geometric Demons for three values of γ. Corresponding fibers in different subjects share colors. **Bottom**: Evolution of the image and fiber similarity measures with varying γ is shown in (d) and (e) (one curve per subject). For each metric, values were scaled using min-max normalization.

As expected, TD improved fiber registration compared to SD. Similarly, GD further improved fiber alignment consistently for all subjects. However, the same set of fibers used for registration was used for performance evaluation. This favors our method as we explicitly optimize a metric evaluated on those fibers. For a fair evaluation, we measured in another experiment the fiber similarity on the 50 bundles that were left aside (100 bundles were extracted and only 50 were kept). In other words, we perform registration on half of the bundles and evaluate the result quality on the other half. Results are shown in Fig. 2 (e). We noticed a similar performance between TD and GD, both improving results obtained by SD. However, GD was only using sparse information from tensors over the set of fibers not being tested: having similar results as TD is thus very promising.

4   Discussion

As expected, GD increased fiber matching compared to the scalar and tensor versions while preserving a good match between images. Interestingly, the algorithm performed even better on images themselves in some subjects. Furthermore, when evaluating algorithm performance on a different set of fibers than those used for registration, we found that GD better registers missing structures

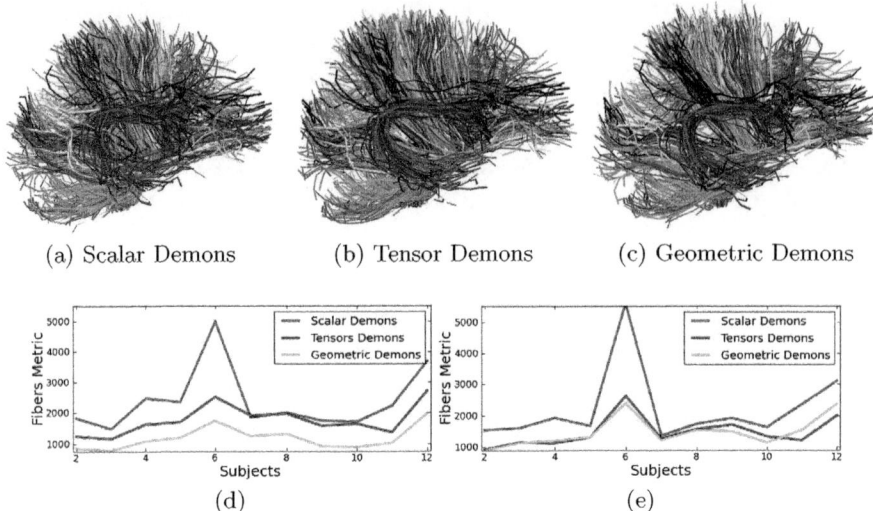

(a) Scalar Demons   (b) Tensor Demons   (c) Geometric Demons

(d)   (e)

Fig. 2. Comparison of Scalar, Tensor and Geometric Demons. Top: Fibers of 11 subjects were overlapped after registering with: (a) Scalar Demons, (b) Tensor Demons, (c) Geometric Demons. Corresponding fibers in subjects share colors. **Bottom:** Fiber similarity metric for each subject and each method evaluated on the fibers set (d) used during registration and (e) left aside.

than SD, and performs similarly to TD. It also shows that a small set of fibers might be sufficient for a proper registration of the white matter across subjects.

By using labeled fibers instead of purely tensor information, we add relevant features that were previously extracted as prior such as region connection or fibers differently classified which should not be merged. Even though the efficacy of trusting fibers is open to discussion, classification of fibers is an active topic in research and we believe this information should not be discarded.

Nevertheless, application of GD to joint T_1/fiber registration can be improved. First, the CPD imposes to have a fiber-to-fiber correspondence. Using [13] we consistently extract corresponding single fiber representatives from subjects, which is not optimal. Indeed, not all bundles can be reduced to a single line. We are working towards using the currents as in [6], which would allow us to directly use sets of lines instead of points. Second, the resampling deformation field had to be inverted to obtain the geometric deformation. A better strategy would be to use the log-domain diffeomorphic Demons [15] which optimizes the logarithm (in the Lie group sense) of the deformation field s: $l = \log(s)$. Then, the inverse field is easily obtained by taking the exponential of the opposite of l.

5   Conclusion

In this work, we presented an extension of the well-established Demons algorithm for non-linear registration taking into account geometric constraints.

The framework is generic in the sense that any type of geometric descriptors, such as line or surfaces, can be incorporated given a differentiable similarity measure.

Within T_1/fiber registration, the GD showed to perform better than their scalar and tensor versions: the obtained deformation field correctly aligns the T_1 images, and also better aligns fibers. This can be used to perform group studies targeting, at the same time, voxel-based morphometry (VBM) and shape analysis of structures of interest: a unique deformation field mapping simultaneously images and structures can be obtained. This gives a consistent framework for analyzing and comparing results between VBM and shape analysis.

As future work we plan to improve the similarity measure between geometric structures, i.e. using currents, and incorporate new structures such as sulcal lines or cortical surfaces. Another application is the combined registration and clustering of fibers: increased fiber registration can help clustering algorithms, which can in turn guide the registration.

Acknowledgements. This work was supported by the ANR (Agence Nationale de la Recherche) "programme blanc" KaraMetria number ANR-09-BLAN-0332-01.

References

1. Thirion, J.P.: Image matching as a diffusion process: an analogy with Maxwell's demons. Medical Image Analysis 2(3), 243–260 (1998)
2. Beg, M.F., et al.: Computing large deformation metric mappings via geodesic flows of diffeomorphisms. IJCV 61(2), 139–157 (2005)
3. Rueckert, D., Aljabar, P., Heckemann, R.A., Hajnal, J.V., Hammers, A.: Diffeomorphic registration using B-splines. In: Larsen, R., Nielsen, M., Sporring, J. (eds.) MICCAI 2006. LNCS, vol. 4191, pp. 702–709. Springer, Heidelberg (2006)
4. Zhang, H., et al.: Deformable registration of diffusion tensor mr images with explicit orientation optimization. Medical Image Analysis 10(5), 764–785 (2006)
5. Yeo, B., et al.: Dt-refind: Diffusion tensor registration with exact finite-strain differential. IEEE Trans. Med. Imaging 28(12), 1914–1928 (2009)
6. Durrleman, S., et al.: Registration, atlas estimation and variability analysis of white matter fiber bundles modeled as currents. NeuroImage 55(3), 1073–1090 (2011)
7. Yeo, B., et al.: Spherical demons: Fast diffeomorphic landmark-free surface registration. IEEE Trans. Med. Imaging 29(3), 650–668 (2010)
8. Auzias, G., et al.: Diffeomorphic brain registration under exhaustive sulcal constraints. IEEE Trans. Med. Imaging (January 2011)
9. Ha, L.K., et al.: Image registration driven by combined probabilistic and geometric descriptors. In: Jiang, T., Navab, N., Pluim, J.P.W., Viergever, M.A. (eds.) MICCAI 2010. LNCS, vol. 6362, pp. 602–609. Springer, Heidelberg (2010)
10. Sotiras, A., et al.: Simultaneous geometric - iconic registration. In: Jiang, T., Navab, N., Pluim, J.P.W., Viergever, M.A. (eds.) MICCAI 2010. LNCS, vol. 6362, pp. 676–683. Springer, Heidelberg (2010)
11. Vercauteren, T., et al.: Diffeomorphic demons: Efficient non-parametric image registration. NeuroImage 45(sup.1), S61–S72 (2009)

12. Poupon, C., et al.: A database dedicated to anatomo-functional study of human brain connectivity. In: 12th HBM Neuroimage, Florence, Italie, vol. (646) (2006)
13. Guevara, P., et al.: Robust clustering of massive tractography datasets. Neuroimage 54(3), 1975–1993 (2011)
14. Fillard, P., et al.: Clinical DT-MRI estimation, smoothing and fiber tracking with log-Euclidean metrics. IEEE Trans. Med. Imaging 26(11), 1472–1482 (2007)
15. Vercauteren, T., et al.: Symmetric log-domain diffeomorphic registration: A demons-based approach. In: Metaxas, D., Axel, L., Fichtinger, G., Székely, G. (eds.) MICCAI 2008, Part I. LNCS, vol. 5241, pp. 754–761. Springer, Heidelberg (2008)

Improving Registration Using Multi-channel Diffeomorphic Demons Combined with Certainty Maps

Daniel Forsberg[1,2,3], Yogesh Rathi[4], Sylvain Bouix[4], Demian Wassermann[4], Hans Knutsson[2,3], and Carl-Fredrik Westin[5]

[1] Sectra Imtec, Linköping, Sweden
[2] Department of Biomedical Engineering, Linköping University, Sweden
[3] Center for Medical Image Science and Visualization (CMIV),
Linköping University, Sweden
[4] Psychiatry Neuroimaging Laboratory, Brigham and Womens Hospital,
Harvard Medical School, Boston, MA, USA
[5] Laboratory of Mathematics in Imaging, Brigham and Womens Hospital,
Harvard Medical School, Boston, MA, USA

Abstract. The number of available imaging modalities increases both in clinical practice and in clinical studies. Even though data from multiple modalities might be available, image registration is typically only performed using data from a single modality. In this paper, we propose using certainty maps together with multi-channel diffeomorphic demons in order to improve both accuracy and robustness when performing image registration. The proposed method is evaluated using DTI data, multiple region overlap measures and a fiber bundle similarity metric.

1 Introduction

Image registration is a well-known concept within the medical image domain and has proven to be useful in a number of situations and applications. The basic idea of image registration is to find a displacement field d that aligns a source image S with a target image T. The research related to image registration is vast and the available methods are many [4]. However, up until today, most research regarding image registration has been related to scalar image registration, although there has been a constant increase of available imaging modalities both for clinical practice and clinical studies. Often each modality has its own unique and, thus, complementary information depicting the underlying anatomy, see Fig. 1 for an example of this. Thus, combining multiple modalities and performing multi-variate image registration is likely to improve both accuracy and robustness.

The primary challenge in registration of multi-variate data lies in finding a suitable way of fusing information from different modalities. The first approach for multi-variate image registration is to expand scalar similarity metrics to their corresponding multi-variate versions, e.g. multi-variate mutual information. However, the computational costs associated with estimating multi-variate

T. Liu et al. (Eds.): MBIA 2011, LNCS 7012, pp. 19–26, 2011.

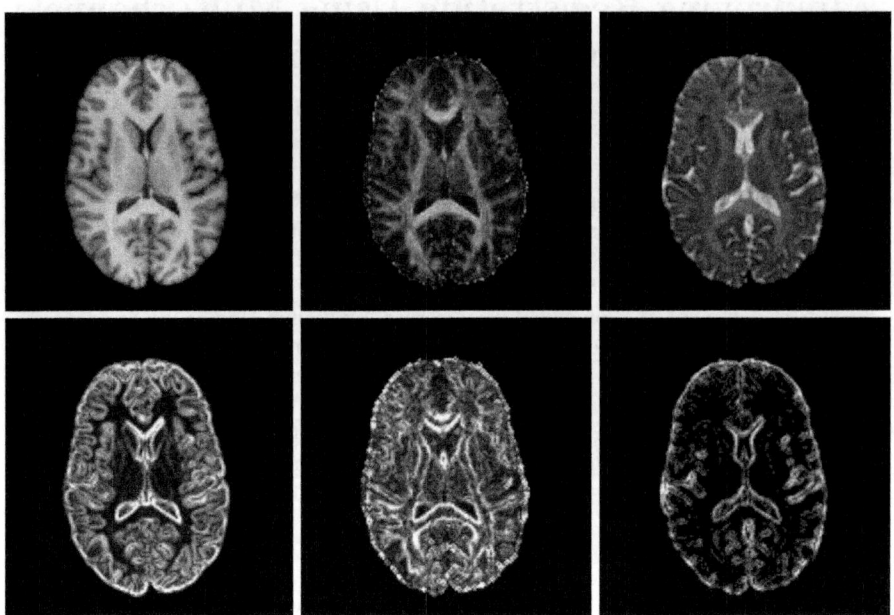

Fig. 1. Comparing a T1 image with images depicting fractional anisotropy and parallel diffusivity reveals the complimentary information provided by different modalities. This becomes more apparent when observing the gradient of the corresponding images and especially in regards of white matter and gray matter.

mutual information makes it too cumbersome to use and calls for different assumptions or approximations to be made [11,12].

A common approach is to fuse the information from the multi-variate data into a single scalar, typically done for diffusion tensor imaging (DTI) data where fractional anisotropy (FA) is used, and then to apply standard scalar-based registration methods. Li and Verma [7] introduced a novel multi-channel method, which contrary to fusing multi-variate data at image/intensity level, instead fuses information on a feature level. Another novelty in their suggestion is that they use independent component analysis and a choose-max approach to fuse and extract relevant information.

Another approach is to use multi-channel registration. Typically, an arbitrary number of channels can be used with arbitrary scalar valued images in each channel (e.g. intensity values, scalar values derived from the tensor or feature values). This approach was explored by Guimond *et al.* and by Park*et al.* [3,8], where they used a multi-channel registration method primarily influenced by the demons algorithm. Avant *et al.* [1] presented the method multi-variate symmetric normalization (MVSyN), which is an extension of the SyN registration method to handle multiple channels. In common for these methods, is that each channel independently estimates an update field for each variate, which are then simply averaged to update the full displacement field.

In this paper we expand a multi-channel version of the well-known demons algorithm to also include certainties of the channel-wise estimated update fields, in order to create a spatially adaptive combination of the update fields by use of weighted averaging. The multi-channel registration is compared with single channel registration on a set of DTI data using various metrics for region overlap and a metric for fiber bundle similarity.

2 Multi-channel Diffemorphic Demons with Weighted Averaging

The demons algorithm was introduced by Thirion in 1995 [13] and has since then gone through a number of evolutionary steps, where one of the more recent is the extension of demons to include diffeomorphic deformations [14]. The basic diffeomorphic demons can be explained as follows:

1. Set $d = 0$ and let $D = S \circ d$.
2. Estimate an update field u as:

$$u = \frac{(D - T)\,\nabla T}{\nabla T^2 + (D - T)^2}$$

3. If fluid regularization, update u with $u * g_{fluid}$.
4. Add u to displacement field d using compositive field accumulation and the exponential update field (ensures a diffeomorphic deformation):

$$d = d \circ \exp(u)$$

5. If elastic regularization, update d with $d * g_{elastic}$.
6. Update D.

$$D = S \circ d$$

7. Repeat step 2-6 until convergence.

The demons has previously been extended to handle multi-variate data, see [3,9]. The suggestion by Guimond *et al.* is somewhat *ad hoc*, where the update fields are simply averaged between the different channels, whereas the suggestion by Peyrat *et al.* is more formally derived but where the resulting solution is rather similar.

2.1 Incorporating Local Certainty

In this work we will use the suggestion by Guimond *et al.* to average the update fields of the different channels, but we will extend their suggestion with the use of channel-specific certainty maps, in order to replace the standard averaging with weighted averaging. Thus, step 2, in the above description, will be replaced with the following sub-steps:

- Estimate an update field u_i for each channel coupled with a certainty c_i:

$$u_i = \frac{(D_i - T_i)\,\nabla T_i}{\nabla T_i^2 + (D_i - T_i)^2}$$

$$c_i = \|\nabla T_i^T \nabla T_i\|$$

- Normalize the certainty c_i.

$$\hat{c}_i = \frac{c_i}{\max c_i}$$

- Employ weighted averaging to the channel-specific update fields using their respective certainty maps.

$$u = \frac{\sum_i \hat{c}_i u_i}{\sum_i \hat{c}_i}$$

The reason for using weighted averaging is to allow channels with high certainty to dominate the combination of the channel-specific update fields, instead of just averaging them. The usefulness of incorporating certainty into various signal/image processing operations has been shown earlier, e.g. normalized convolution by Knutsson and Westin [5]. Some examples of utilizing image registration can be found in work by Kybic and by Risholm et al. [6,10], however, the usage of certainty in image registration remains sparse. In case of the demons, and as in the case of many other registration algorithms, the reliability of the update field is usually the highest where the structural content is high, hence, we suggest to use the norm of structure tensor as certainty measure, here estimated as the outer product of the gradient.

3   Experiments and Results

3.1   Evaluation Metrics

Evaluating image registration is a non-trivial task because of the lack of a gold standard. A single metric can seldom capture all aspects of a successful registration. Therefore, in this paper we make use of a number of different metrics, evaluating various aspects of the registration results.

The overall registration accuracy of the brain is evaluated using two overlap measures, quantifying how well the labeled source and target volumes overlap with each other. The first measure is target overlap (TO), which is the intersection between similarly labeled regions r in S and T divided by the volume of the regions in T.

$$TO = \frac{\sum_r |T_r \cap S_r|}{\sum_r |T_r|}$$

where $\|$ denotes the volume in voxels. The second measure is union overlap UO, which is the intersection of S_r and T_r over their union.

$$UO = \frac{\sum_r |T_r \cap S_r|}{\sum_r |T_r \cup S_r|}$$

To complement these agreement measures, false negative and false positive errors were also computed. For a given region r, a false negative error FN is a measure of how much of the target region that has been missed. The false negative error is given as the volume of the target region outside of the source region divided by the volume of the target region.

$$FN = \frac{\sum_r |T_r \setminus S_r|}{\sum_r |T_r|}$$

A false positive error FP, on the other hand, measures how much of the volume outside the target region that has been incorrectly labeled as a part of the region. This is given as the volume of the source region outside of the corresponding target region divided by the volume of the source region.

$$FP = \frac{\sum_r |S_r \setminus T_r|}{\sum_r |S_r|}$$

To better evaluate the registration in terms of fiber tracts, since we are using DTI data, we utilize a similarity measure developed by Wassermann et al. [16], where each fiber tract is blurred using Gaussian Processes. Based upon the blurred fibers, it is possible to create a representation of the fiber bundles for which an inner product between two fiber bundles F and F' can be defined, $< F, F' >$. With an inner product defined, a fiber bundle similarity measure, ranging from 0 to 1, is easily constructed as:

$$< F, F' >_N = \frac{< F, F' >}{\|F\|\|F'\|}$$

where

$$\|F\|^2 = < F, F >$$

3.2   Data Acquisition

The data consisted of 10 healthy subjects, where diffusion weighted images (DWI) scans had been previously acquired on a 3-T GE system using an echo planar imaging (EPI) DWI sequence. The following scan parameters were used: TR 17000 ms, TE 78 ms, FOV 24 cm, 144x144 encoding steps, 1.7 mm slice thickness. All scans had 85 axial slices parallel to the ACPC line covering the whole brain. Along with DWI images, T1 and T2 images were also acquired.

3.3   Data Pre-prcessing

The scalar DTI measures fractional anisotropy (FA) and parallel diffusivity (PD) where estimated from the DWI data.

The labeling of different brain regions (180 different cortical and subcortical regions) was achieved using the Freesurfer software[1]. A T2 image, which was in

---

[1] surfer.nmr.mgh.harvard.edu

the same coordinate space as the T1 image, was then diffeomorphically registered to the baseline ($S0$) diffusion weighted image of the same subject using FSL software's nonlinear image registration tool (FNIRT). The obtained transform was applied to the T1 image and the label map, to obtain a T1 image and a label map in the coordinate space of the diffusion images.

The tractography was done using the Slicer software[2], where corpus callosum of each subject was handsegmented and then used as seeding points for standard single-tensor tractography.

3.4   Evaluation

To evaluate the suggested method, one subject was selected as target and the nine remaining subjects where then individually registered to the target subject. The obtained displacement fields were applied to the labels maps and the fiber bundles. The deformed label maps and fiber bundles were then compared with the target's label map and fiber bundle, using the previously described metrics. The evaluation was done using both single channel T1 and FA, multi-channel T1/FA and T1/FA/PD registration.

The results of the evaluation are presented in Table 1 and are easy to interpret, multi-channel image registration with weighted averaging improves both accuracy and robustness, albeit the improvements cannot considered to be significant. Example slices of the results are depicted in Fig. 2.

Table 1. Summary of the results from the evaluation of multi-channel registration. The results are consistently showing better accuracy and robustness for multi-channel registration, albeit minor.

Channel combination	TO	UO	FN	FP	$< F_T, F_D >$
T1	0.50 ± 0.06	0.34 ± 0.05	0.50 ± 0.06	0.50 ± 0.06	0.52 ± 0.12
FA	0.47 ± 0.04	0.31 ± 0.04	0.53 ± 0.04	0.52 ± 0.05	0.55 ± 0.09
T1 and FA	0.52 ± 0.05	0.35 ± 0.04	0.48 ± 0.05	0.48 ± 0.05	0.55 ± 0.12
T1, FA and PD	0.52 ± 0.04	0.35 ± 0.04	0.48 ± 0.05	0.48 ± 0.04	0.55 ± 0.12

4   Discussion

It is interesting to note that these results are similar to the ones achieved by Guimond et al. and by Park et al. [3,8] where they observed an improvement when using a multi-channel demons registration but without showing it to be significant. The same can be found in [1]. In this context it also worth noting that, in a recent evaluation of various registration algorithms on DTI data [15], using both single-variate and multi-variate registration methods, the single-variate methods often performed on the same level and sometimes even better than the multi-variate methods.

---

[2] www.slicer.org

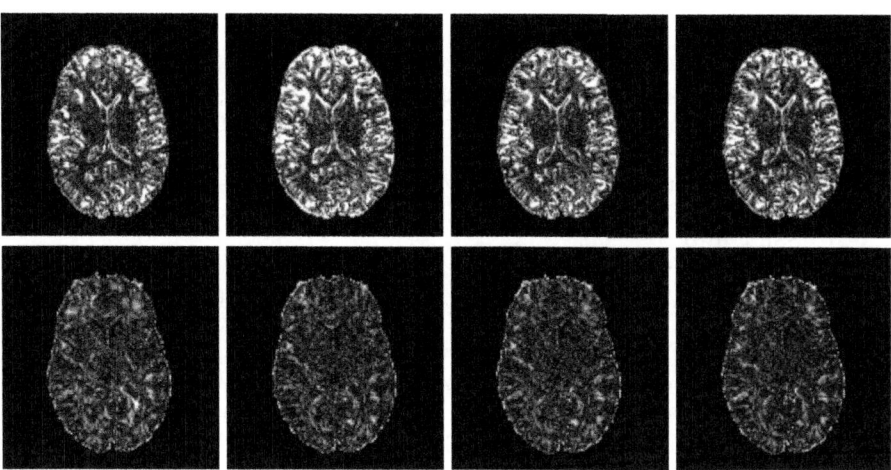

Fig. 2. Absolute difference of target and deformed T1 (top row) and FA (bottom row) slices using (from left) single channel T1 and FA, and multi-channel T1/FA and T1/FA/PD registration. Although the differences are not large, it can be observed that the multi-channel solutions performs better than the single channel solutions.

In order to improve the results, various approaches were attempted, such as; changing certainty measure (magnitude of the gradient), adding a sigmoid mapping of the certainty and relaxing the regularization. In our experiments, the relaxing of the regularization showed the greatest impact. The difference between the single-channel and multi-channel increased when removing the diffeomorphic constraint but to the cost of a very irregular deformation and was therefore refrained from. A possible remedy here, would be to employ adaptive anisotropic regularization instead of isotropic Gaussian regularization [2].

A justified question at this moment, is whether multi-channel registration adds something significant to the end result or not. As the results in this paper and in [1,3,8] show a consistent improvement when utilizing multi-channel registration it is reasonable to argue that multi-channel registration is valuable, however, when fusing the information more elaborate approaches must be chosen, e.g. along the line of the Li and Verma's proposal in [7].

Future works includes evaluating the combination of adaptive anisotropic regularization together with multi-channel image registration, and exploring more elaborate ways to fuse the information of multiple channels

Acknowledgement. Support for this research was provided in part by the Swedish Research Council (2007-4786), AgoraLink at Linköping University and the National Institute of Health (R01MH082918, R01MH074794, R01MH092862, P41RR013218).

References

1. Avants, B., Duda, J., Zhang, H., Gee, J.: Multivariate normalization with symmetric diffeomorphisms for multivariate studies. In: Ayache, N., Ourselin, S., Maeder, A. (eds.) MICCAI 2007, Part I. LNCS, vol. 4791, pp. 359–366. Springer, Heidelberg (2007)
2. Forsberg, D., Andersson, M., Knutsson, H.: Adaptive anisotropic regularization of deformation fields for non-rigid registration using the morphon framework. In: ICASSP (2010)
3. Guimond, A., Guttmann, C., Warfield, S., Westin, C.F.: Deformable registration of DT-MRI data based on transformation invariant tensor characteristics. In: ISBI (2002)
4. Holden, M.: A Review of Geometric Transformations for Nonrigid Body Registration. IEEE Transactions on Medical Imaging (2008)
5. Knutsson, H., Westin, C.F.: Normalized and Differential Convolution: Methods for Interpolation and Filtering of Incomplete and Uncertain Data. In: CVPR (1993)
6. Kybic, J.: Bootstrap resampling for image registration uncertainty estimation without ground truth. IEEE Transactions on Image Processing (2010)
7. Li, Y., Verma, R.: Multichannel Image Registration by Feature-Based Information Fusion. IEEE Transactions on Medical Imaging (2011)
8. Park, H.J., Kubicki, M., Shenton, M.E., Guimond, A., McCarley, R.W., Maier, S.E., Kikinis, R., Jolesz, F.A., Westin, C.F.: Spatial Normalization of Diffusion Tensor MRI Using Multiple Channels. Neuroimage (2003)
9. Peyrat, J.-M., Delingette, H., Sermesant, M., Pennec, X., Xu, C., Ayache, N.: Registration of 4D time-series of cardiac images with multichannel diffeomorphic demons. In: Metaxas, D., Axel, L., Fichtinger, G., Székely, G. (eds.) MICCAI 2008, Part II. LNCS, vol. 5242, pp. 972–979. Springer, Heidelberg (2008)
10. Risholm, P., Pieper, S., Samset, E., Wells III, W.M.: Summarizing and visualizing uncertainty in non-rigid registration. In: Jiang, T., Navab, N., Pluim, J.P.W., Viergever, M.A. (eds.) MICCAI 2010. LNCS, vol. 6362, pp. 554–561. Springer, Heidelberg (2010)
11. Rohde, G.K., Pajevic, S., Pierpaoli, C., Basser, P.J.: A comprehensive approach for multi-channel image registration. In: Gee, J.C., Maintz, J.B.A., Vannier, M.W. (eds.) WBIR 2003. LNCS, vol. 2717, pp. 214–223. Springer, Heidelberg (2003)
12. Studholme, C.: Incorporating DTI data as a constraint in deformation tensor morphometry between T1 MR images. In: Karssemeijer, N., Lelieveldt, B. (eds.) IPMI 2007. LNCS, vol. 4584, pp. 223–232. Springer, Heidelberg (2007)
13. Thirion, J.P.: Fast Non-Rigid Matching of 3D Medical Images. Research Report RR-2547, INRIA (1995)
14. Vercauteren, T., Pennec, X., Perchant, A., Ayache, N.: Non-parametric diffeomorphic image registration with the demons algorithm. In: Ayache, N., Ourselin, S., Maeder, A. (eds.) MICCAI 2007, Part II. LNCS, vol. 4792, pp. 319–326. Springer, Heidelberg (2007)
15. Wang, Y., Gupta, A., Liu, Z., Zhang, H., Escolar, M., Gilmore, J., Gouttard, S., Fillard, P., Maltbie, E., Gerig, G., Styner, M.: Dti registration in atlas based fiber analysis of infantile krabbe disease. Neuroimage (2011)
16. Wassermann, D., Bloy, L., Kanterakis, E., Verma, R., Deriche, R.: Unsupervised white matter fiber clustering and tract probability map generation: Applications of a Gaussian process framework for white matter fibers. NeuroImage (2010)

Identifying Neuroimaging and Proteomic Biomarkers for MCI and AD via the Elastic Net

Li Shen[1,*], Sungeun Kim[1], Yuan Qi[2], Mark Inlow[1,3], Shanker Swaminathan[1], Kwangsik Nho[1], Jing Wan[1], Shannon L. Risacher[1], Leslie M. Shaw[4], John Q. Trojanowski[4], Michael W. Weiner[5], Andrew J. Saykin[1,*], and ADNI

[1] Radiology and Imaging Sciences, Indiana University, IN, USA
[2] Computer Science, Statistics and Biology, Purdue University, IN, USA
[3] Mathematics, Rose-Hulman Institute of Technology, IN, USA
[4] Pathology and Laboratory Medicine, University of Pennsylvania, PA, USA
[5] Radiology, Medicine and Psychiatry, UC San Francisco, CA, USA

Abstract. Multi-modal neuroimaging and biomarker data provide exciting opportunities to enhance our understanding of phenotypic characteristics associated with complex disorders. This study focuses on integrative analysis of structural MRI data and proteomic data from an RBM panel to examine their predictive power and identify relevant biomarkers in a large MCI/AD cohort. MRI data included volume and thickness measures of 98 regions estimated by FreeSurfer. RBM data included 146 proteomic analytes extracted from plasma and serum. A sparse learning model, elastic net logistic regression, was proposed to classify AD and MCI, and select disease-relevant biomarkers. A linear support vector machine coupled with feature selection was employed for comparison. Combining RBM and MRI data yielded improved prediction rates: HC vs AD (91.9%), HC vs MCI (90.5%) and MCI vs AD (86.5%). Elastic net identified a small set of meaningful imaging and proteomic biomarkers. The elastic net has great power to optimize the sparsity of feature selection while maintaining high predictive power. Its application to multi-modal imaging and biomarker data has considerable potential for discovering biomarkers and enhancing mechanistic understanding of AD and MCI.

1 Introduction

Multi-modal neuroimaging data, such as magnetic resonance imaging (MRI) and positron emission tomography (PET), studied independently or coupled with other biomarker data (e.g., cerebrospinal fluid (CSF) and neuropsychological assessments), have been shown to be sensitive to Alzheimer's Disease (AD) and mild cognitive impairment (MCI, thought to be the prodromal stage of AD). Although recent studies reported promising prediction rates by integrating these

* Correspondence to L Shen (shenli@iupui.edu) or AJ Saykin (asaykin@iupui.edu). Data collection and sharing for this project was funded by the Alzheimer's Disease Neuroimaging Initiative (ADNI) (U01 AG024904, http://adni.loni.ucla.edu). This project was also supported by NIA 1RC 2AG036535, NIA P30 AG10133, NIA R01 AG19771, CTSI-IUSM/CTR(RR025761), NSF-IIS 1117335, and NSF-IIS 1054903.

T. Liu et al. (Eds.): MBIA 2011, LNCS 7012, pp. 27–34, 2011.
© Springer-Verlag Berlin Heidelberg 2011

multi-modal data [7,10,16], few were focused on identifying a small set of disease relevant biomarkers [13] to enhance our understanding of phenotypic character-istics and underlying mechanisms associated with complex disorders.

With these observations, this paper has the following aims: (1) investigate the predictive power of a new set of proteomic analytes from an RBM panel, (2) study whether or not combining structural MRI and proteomic data can enhance prediction rates, and (3) employ a principled sparse learning method, elastic net logistic regression [5], in the study to maximize prediction accuracy while optimizing the selection of disease sensitive biomarkers. Our overarching goal is to construct from multimodal data sparse models which combine ease of interpretation with high predictive power. The results may provide important information about potential surrogate biomarkers for therapeutic trials.

2   Materials and Methods

Data used in this study were obtained from the Alzheimer's Disease Neuroimag-ing Initiative (ADNI) database (adni.loni.ucla.edu). ADNI is a landmark in-vestigation sponsored by the NIH and industrial partners designed to collect longitudinal neuroimaging, biological and clinical information from over 800 par-ticipants that will track the neural correlates of memory loss from an early stage. The following data from 819 ADNI participants were downloaded from the ADNI database: all baseline 1.5 T MRI scans, the RBM (Rules-Based Medicine) mul-tiplex proteomic analytes extracted from plasma and serum, and demographic and baseline diagnosis information. Further information can be found in [15] and at www.adni-info.org. For one baseline scan of each participant, FreeSurfer V4 was employed to automatically label cortical and subcortical tissue classes [3,4] and to extract target region volume and cortical thickness, as well as to extract total intracranial volume (ICV). For each hemisphere, thickness measures of 34 cortical regions of interest (ROIs) and volume measures of 15 cortical and sub-cortical ROIs (Fig. 1) were included in this study. Using the regression weights derived from the healthy participants, all the FreeSurfer measures were adjusted for the baseline age, gender, education, handedness, and ICV, and all the RBM proteomic measures were adjusted for the baseline age, gender, education and handedness. 551 out of 819 participants (57 healthy control (HC), 388 MCI, 106 AD participants) had both FreeSurfer and RBM data available. To have a bal-anced data set among different diagnostic groups, we included all HC and AD participants and a randomly selected set of 110 (out of 388) MCI participants in this study. Their characteristics are summarized in Table 1.

Elastic Net: Elastic net logistic regression is a regularized version of logistic regression designed to provide good classification performance while employing a minimal number of predictor variables. Let $y_i \in \{0, 1\}$ denote the class mem-bership of the ith observation and let X_i denote the corresponding vector of p classification variables. Elastic net logistic regression uses the standard logistic regression model for the dependence of Y on X:

$$\Pr(Y = 1 | X) = \frac{1}{1 + e^{-(\beta_0 + X^T \beta)}}, \qquad \Pr(Y = 0 | X) = \frac{1}{1 + e^{+(\beta_0 + X^T \beta)}}.$$

Table 1. Participant characteristics

Category	HC	MCI	AD	p-value
Gender (M/F)	30/27	60/50	60/46	0.88
Handedness (R/L)	53/4	104/6	99/7	0.91
Baseline Age (years, mean±SD)	75.2±5.8	75.0±7.4	74.8±8.1	0.95
Education (years, mean±SD)	15.7±2.7	15.5±3.0	15.1±3.3	0.37
ICV (cm^3, mean±SD)	1506±143	1559±169	1558±195	0.13

However, in order to produce sparse classification weight vectors, it estimates β by the maximizer of the penalized logistic regression log likelihood function

$$\mathcal{L}(\beta_0, \beta) = \frac{1}{n} \sum_{i=1}^{n} \{y_i(\beta_0 + X_i^T \beta) - \log(1 + e^{(\beta_0 + X_i^T \beta)})\} - \lambda P_\alpha(\beta)$$

in which $P_\alpha(\beta) = \alpha \sum_{j=1}^{p} |\beta(j)| + (1-\alpha) \sum_{j=1}^{p} \{\beta(j)\}^2$ is the elastic net penalty. Note that this penalty function is a convex combination of the L_1 lasso penalty and the L_2 ridge regression penalty. By providing a smooth trade-off between these two penalties, elastic net penalization capitalizes on the strengths of both while minimizing their weaknesses; see Friedman et al [5] for additional details. The imaging and proteomic biomarker data was analyzed using the implementation of elastic net logistic regression provided in the Matlab package glmnet.

Experimental Setting: The elastic net is in essence a linear classifier, where logistic regression is just a procedural step. For a fair comparison, a linear support vector machine (SVM) [14] coupled with a widely used feature selection scheme (SVM-based Recursive Feature Elimination, or SVM-RFE [6]) was applied in this study. The LIBSVM toolbox was employed to implement SVM and SVM-RFE using a linear kernel with default setting. We ran SVM-RFE using the training data only to select the top $n\%$ features and then trained a SVM classifier using these features only. We tested $n = 10, 25$ and 100, and denoted the corresponding procedures as SVM_{10}, SVM_{25} and SVM (i.e., SVM_{100}, equivalent to no feature selection), respectively. For the elastic net, we did three experiments with $\alpha = 0.25, 0.5$ and 0.75 (to adjust the amount of ridge and lasso), respectively, and the parameter λ was tuned by a 10-fold cross-validation procedure using the training data only. These experiments were applied to three data sets: (1) FreeSurfer data (98 variables), (2) RBM data (146 variables), and (3) combined FreeSurfer and RBM data (244 variables, a simple concatenation of the two modalities). Prediction accuracy was estimated using 5-fold cross-validation.

3   Results

We use EN25, EN50 and EN75 to indicate the elastic net classifiers with $\alpha = 0.25, 0.5$, and 0.75, respectively. Table 2 summarizes the 5-fold cross-validation results for classifying HC vs AD, HC vs MCI, and MCI vs AD for each combination of six methods (SVM_{10}, SVM_{25}, SVM, EN25, EN50 and EN75) and three

Table 2. Cross validation results (%): mean±SD is shown for accuracy and AUROC

		FreeSurfer (FS)		RBM		Combined FS and RBM	
		Accuracy	AUROC	Accuracy	AUROC	Accuracy	AUROC
HC vs AD	SVM_{10}	82.3 ± 4.1	88.9 ± 4.6	76.4 ± 5.6	84.0 ± 5.9	91.6 ± 4.6	97.0 ± 3.0
	SVM_{25}	83.4 ± 7.4	89.8 ± 5.3	80.6 ± 3.3	87.2 ± 2.6	91.6 ± 5.1	97.1 ± 2.1
	SVM	84.5 ± 9.7	91.9 ± 6.2	80.0 ± 8.4	89.5 ± 4.4	91.9 ± 3.1	96.3 ± 2.4
	EN25	84.7 ± 5.3	94.2 ± 4.8	81.2 ± 3.3	91.8 ± 3.5	91.5 ± 4.2	97.6 ± 2.0
	EN50	85.9 ± 6.0	94.8 ± 4.7	83.5 ± 4.9	90.6 ± 3.7	91.5 ± 4.2	97.1 ± 3.3
	EN75	86.6 ± 6.2	94.6 ± 5.6	83.7 ± 5.1	89.9 ± 3.8	90.9 ± 5.3	97.1 ± 3.6
HC vs MCI	SVM_{10}	70.7 ± 4.7	73.2 ± 8.1	74.9 ± 7.2	84.5 ± 5.0	85.0 ± 4.5	90.9 ± 6.3
	SVM_{25}	65.9 ± 7.4	68.5 ± 10.5	81.5 ± 8.6	91.2 ± 4.2	89.2 ± 3.5	94.9 ± 4.5
	SVM	63.5 ± 10.1	63.7 ± 6.7	87.4 ± 4.4	92.8 ± 4.3	89.1 ± 6.3	93.7 ± 3.7
	EN25	74.3 ± 5.6	79.3 ± 8.3	87.4 ± 3.2	95.3 ± 2.6	89.2 ± 5.3	96.1 ± 3.3
	EN50	73.7 ± 6.2	79.8 ± 8.3	86.8 ± 6.7	94.8 ± 2.9	90.5 ± 7.6	96.0 ± 3.5
	EN75	74.3 ± 6.0	80.8 ± 7.5	84.5 ± 5.1	94.3 ± 3.2	89.9 ± 5.6	95.6 ± 4.0
MCI vs AD	SVM_{10}	62.2 ± 10.3	70.6 ± 12.4	80.9 ± 8.2	86.1 ± 8.1	81.4 ± 5.1	88.7 ± 4.9
	SVM_{25}	61.9 ± 8.3	70.0 ± 8.8	82.3 ± 3.3	89.4 ± 3.1	79.1 ± 8.7	90.1 ± 4.0
	SVM	53.5 ± 7.4	62.2 ± 8.9	80.4 ± 5.3	88.2 ± 5.4	82.8 ± 5.7	91.4 ± 5.5
	EN25	65.5 ± 12.4	72.7 ± 10.6	83.6 ± 6.8	93.0 ± 3.3	84.1 ± 5.7	92.9 ± 4.1
	EN50	66.4 ± 11.9	72.4 ± 11.4	82.7 ± 6.0	93.1 ± 2.7	86.0 ± 3.9	93.3 ± 3.7
	EN75	66.4 ± 13.3	72.4 ± 12.0	83.7 ± 4.0	93.1 ± 2.2	86.5 ± 5.2	94.0 ± 3.1

data sets (FreeSurfer, RBM, combined FreeSurfer and RBM). These results are very encouraging in the following sense: (1) Elastic net classifiers outperformed SVMs in terms of overall accuracy and area under ROC (AUROC) in almost all the cases, while the performances of EN25, EN50 and EN75 did not differ significantly (paired samples test on AUROC $p > 0.06$ in all cases). (2) The best prediction rates using FreeSurfer were 86.6% for HC vs AD and 74.3% for HC vs MCI, comparable with the most recent studies using MRI as predictors [7,13,16]. (3) While FreeSurfer data performed slightly better in classifying HC vs AD than RBM data, the latter had surprisingly greater power to distinguish MCI from HC (87.4%) and AD (83.7%). (4) The combined set consistently outperformed either of FreeSurfer and RBM. While the resulting best prediction rate for HC vs AD (91.9%) was competitive with prior multi-modal studies [7,16], the prediction rates for HC vs MCI (90.5%) and MCI vs AD (86.5%) significantly exceeded results from prior studies that did not use RBM data (e.g., [16]).

Either the SVM or the elastic net classifier can be characterized by a weight vector w, which projects each individual data point (i.e., a feature vector) into a 1-D space to produce a discriminative value. Each weight measures the strength of the contribution of the corresponding feature to the final discriminative value. Elastic net seeks to reduce the number of nonzero weights so that only relevant features contribute to the discriminative value. For consistency, we always visualize negative weights $-w$ so that larger values (red) correspond to lower measurement levels in cases. We show the weight maps (Fig. 1-3) only for the combined set analysis, since single modality analyses yielded similar maps.

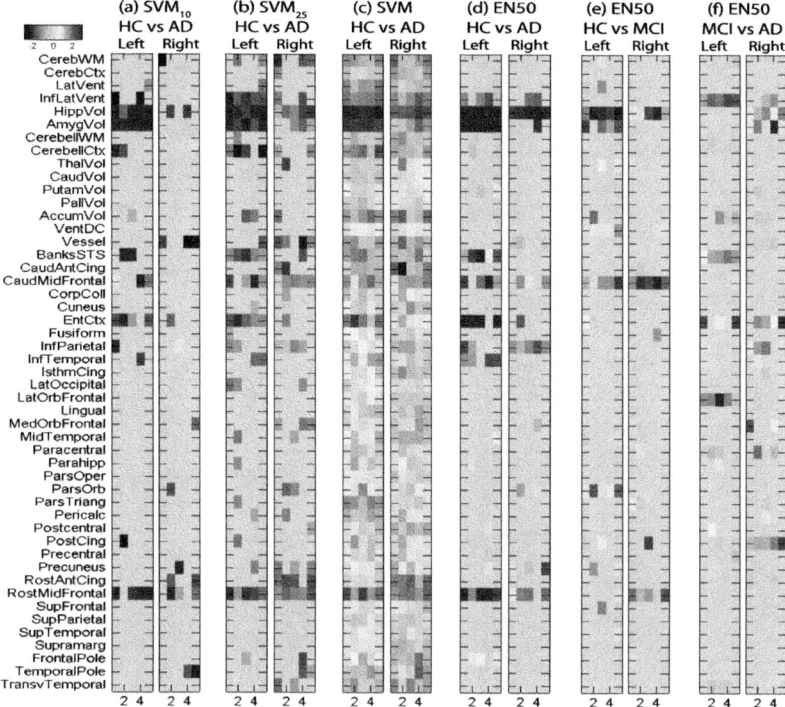

Fig. 1. Heat maps of classifier weights $-w$ for FreeSurfer measures, where weights were plotted against 5 different trials in cross validation tests. Positive values (red) indicate lower measurement levels in cases.

Shown in Fig. 1 are the weights for the FreeSurfer data. Weights for classifying HC vs AD are shown in (a-d) for SVM_{10}, SVM_{25}, SVM and EN50 respectively. While most weights were close to zero, EN50 identified a small number of imaging markers known to be AD-relevant, including hippocampal volume, entorhinal cortex thickness, amygdala volume, and so on. Given many blue blocks (i.e., gray matter increase in AD, which is counter-intuitive), the SVM map was much less sparse and harder to interpret. While SVM_{10} and SVM_{25} identified a few relevant markers similar to EN50, they also yielded some questionable blue blocks and the selected features varied a lot among different cross-validation trials.

Fig. 1(d-f) compare selected features in different classification tasks using EN50. Note that Panels (e,f) selected a smaller number of FreeSurfer features even though the overall prediction accuracies of all three analyses were comparably high. This might imply that the overall prediction accuracies of the latter two tasks (HC vs MCI and MCI vs AD) were more dependent on RBM features than FreeSurfer features. These weights can also be back-projected to the original image space for an intuitive visualization. Fig. 2 shows such a visualization for SVM, EN25 and EN50. EN25 and EN50 yield similar maps that are much more sparse than the SVM map.

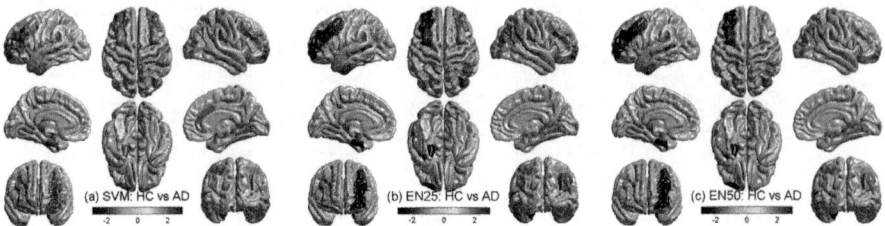

Fig. 2. Back-projection of negative weights $(-w)$ onto cortical surface, where positive values (red) indicate lower measurement levels in cases

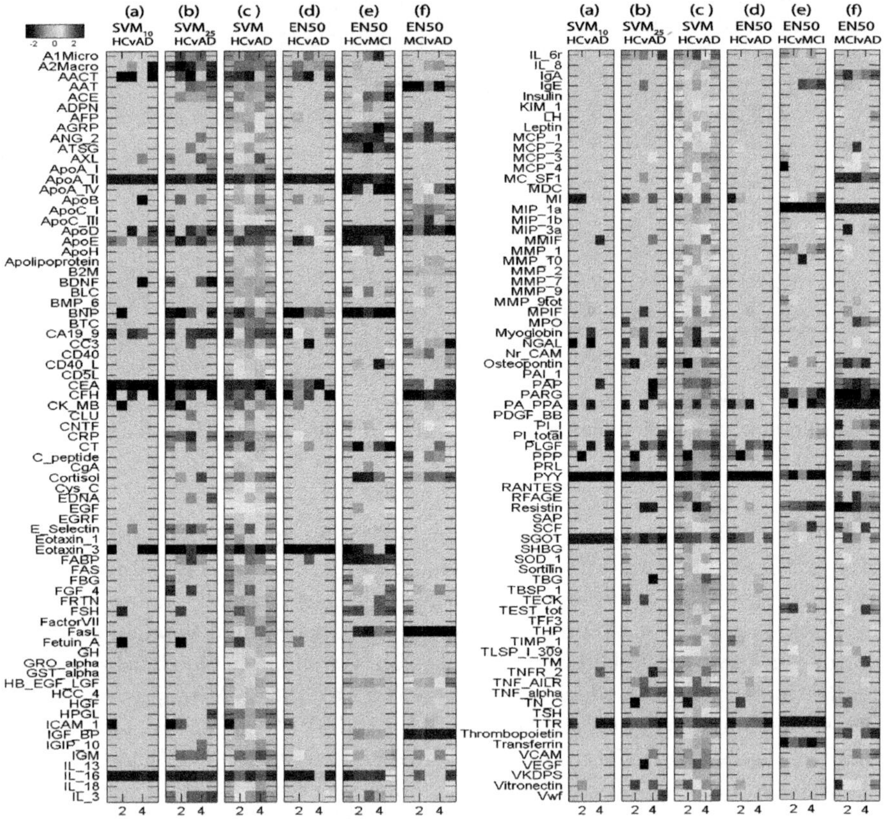

Fig. 3. Heat maps of classifier weights $-w$ for RBM measures, where weights were plotted against 5 different trials in cross validation tests. Positive values (red) indicate lower measurement levels in cases.

Shown in Fig. 3 are the weight maps for RBM features. Again, EN50 yielded fewer relevant features than SVM (see (c-d)). Although SVM_{10} and SVM_{25} (see (a-b)) were able to identify a few interesting features, the selected features varied a lot among different cross-validation trials. Using Elastic Net, a number of RBM analytes were found to have altered concentrations in AD participants compared to HCs. This is consistent with previous studies showing reduced or elevated concentrations of specific analytes in plasma or serum samples of AD participants. The trends for some of the identified analytes follow those in the published literature and are summarized below. Using a similar RBM panel and methodology as done by the ADNI study, O'Bryant et al. identified the analytes alpha-2-macroglobulin (A2Macro), eotaxin 3 (Eotaxin_3) and pancreatic polypeptide (PPP) to be over expressed in the serum of AD participants relative to controls [11] similar to the current findings. Elevated plasma concentrations of complement factor H (CFH) and alpha-2-macroglobulin (A2Macro) [8], reduced plasma concentrations of apolipoprotein AII (ApoA_II) [9] and elevated serum concentration of apolipoprotein B (ApoB) [2] have been observed in AD participants relative to controls, and these were also found in the present study. Apolipoprotein E (ApoE) is a major genetic risk factor for AD [1]. The ApoE concentration in the present study was observed to be reduced in AD participants relative to controls. There are conflicting reports regarding the serum or plasma concentrations of ApoE protein levels in AD, with some studies finding elevated levels, some finding reduced levels and others finding no difference in levels in AD participants relative to controls [12]. Thus its role as a potential AD biomarker is unclear at the present time and needs to be further investigated. A number of novel analytes have also been identified to have altered expression in AD such as carcinoembryonic antigen (CEA) and pregnancy-associated plasma protein A (PA_PPA). These analytes may play a role in disease pathology and warrant further investigation in independent samples. Thus the identification of novel analytes in addition to known analytes demonstrates the power and utility of this approach in identifying potential candidate AD biomarkers.

4   Discussion

We have done an integrative analysis of structural MRI data and proteomic data to examine their predictive power and identify relevant biomarkers in a large MCI/AD cohort. RBM data showed high predictive power to separate MCI from HC and AD. Combining RBM and MRI data yielded further improved prediction rates: HC vs AD (91.9%), HC vs MCI (90.5%) and MCI vs AD (86.5%), which were competitive to or better than similar prior studies. The sparse models generated by elastic net identified a small set of meaningful imaging and proteomic biomarkers and were much easier to interpret than SVM-based models. The elastic net has great power to optimize the sparsity of feature selection while maintaining high predictive power. Its application to multi-modal imaging and biomarker data has considerable potential for discovering biomarkers and enhancing mechanistic understanding of AD and MCI.

Many identified RBM markers warrant further investigation. Replication in independent large samples will be important to confirm these findings. Pathway analysis could be performed as a future direction to identify underlying biological pathways of relevant genes and proteins. This work was focused on sparse linear classifiers applied to the simple concatenation of multi-modal data, since our major goal was to yield easily interpretable models while maintaining high predictive power. An initial analysis of applying SVM with a radial basis function kernel to the same data yielded comparable or less accurate results, and these nonlinear models were much harder to interpret. An interesting future topic is to investigate whether these nonlinear models can help improve the prediction rates as well as derive biologically meaningful results. Another future direction is to apply multi-kernel learning methods (e.g., [7,16]) and see if better predictive models can be achieved and relevant biomarkers can be identified.

References

1. Bertram, L., McQueen, M.B., et al.: Systematic meta-analyses of Alzheimer disease genetic association studies: the AlzGene database. Nat. Genet. 39(1), 17–23 (2007)
2. Caramelli, P., Nitrini, R., et al.: Increased apolipoprotein B serum concentration in Alzheimer's disease. Acta Neurol. Scand. 100(1), 61–63 (1999)
3. Dale, A., Fischl, B., Sereno, M.: Cortical surface-based analysis. I: Segmentation and surface reconstruction. Neuroimage 9(2), 179–194 (1999)
4. Fischl, B., Sereno, M., Dale, A.: Cortical surface-based analysis. II: Inflation, flattening, and a surface-based coordinate system. Neuroimage 9(2), 195–207 (1999)
5. Friedman, J., Hastie, T., Tibshirani, R.: Regularized paths for generalized linear models via coordinate descent. Journal of Statistical Software 33(1) (2010)
6. Guyon, I., Weston, J., Barnhill, S., Vapnik, V.: Gene selection for cancer classification using support vector machines. Machine Learning 46, 389–422 (2002)
7. Hinrichs, C., Singh, V., et al.: Predictive markers for AD in a multi-modality framework: An analysis of MCI progression in the ADNI population. Neuroimage 55(2), 574–589 (2011)
8. Hye, A., Lynham, S., et al.: Proteome-based plasma biomarkers for Alzheimer's disease. Brain 129(Pt 11), 3042–3050 (2006)
9. Kawano, M., Kawakami, M., et al.: Marked decrease of plasma apolipoprotein AI and AII in Japanese patients with late-onset non-familial Alzheimer's disease. Clin. Chim. Acta 239(2), 209–211 (1995)
10. Kloppel, S., Stonnington, C.M., et al.: Automatic classification of MR scans in Alzheimer's disease. Brain 131(Pt 3), 681–689 (2008)
11. O'Bryant, S.E., Xiao, G., et al.: A serum protein-based algorithm for the detection of Alzheimer disease. Arch. Neurol. 67(9), 1077–1081 (2010)
12. Schneider, P., Hampel, H., Buerger, K.: Biological marker candidates of Alzheimer's disease in blood, plasma, and serum. CNS Neurosci. Ther. 15(4), 358–374 (2009)
13. Shen, L., Qi, Y., Kim, S., Nho, K., Wan, J., Risacher, S.L., Saykin, A.J., ADNI: Sparse bayesian learning for identifying imaging biomarkers in AD prediction. In: Jiang, T., Navab, N., Pluim, J.P.W., Viergever, M.A. (eds.) MICCAI 2010. LNCS, vol. 6363, pp. 611–618. Springer, Heidelberg (2010)
14. Vapnik, V.: Statistical Learning Theory. John Wiley and Sons, Chichester (1998)
15. Weiner, M.W., Aisen, P.S., et al.: The Alzheimer's disease neuroimaging initiative: progress report and future plans. Alzheimers Dement 6(3), 202–211e7 (2010)
16. Zhang, D., Wang, Y., et al.: Multimodal classification of Alzheimer's disease and mild cognitive impairment. Neuroimage 55(3), 856–867 (2011)

Heritability of White Matter Fiber Tract Shapes: A HARDI Study of 198 Twins[*]

Yan Jin[1], Yonggang Shi[1], Shantanu H. Joshi[1], Neda Jahanshad[1], Liang Zhan[1], Greig I. de Zubicaray[2], Katie L. McMahon[2], Nicholas G. Martin[3], Margaret J. Wright[3], Arthur W. Toga[1], and Paul M. Thompson[1]

[1] Laboratory of Neuro Imaging, Department of Neurology, School of Medicine, University of California, Los Angeles, CA 90095, USA
[2] fMRI Laboratory, University of Queensland, Brisbane St. Lucia, QLD 4072, Australia
[3] Queensland Institute of Medical Research, Herston, QLD 4029, Australia
{yan.jin,yonggang.shi,shantanu.joshi,neda.jahanshad,
liang.zhan}@loni.ucla.edu,
{greig.dezubicaray,katie.mcmahon}@uq.edu.au,
{nick.martin,margiew}@qimr.edu.au,
{toga,thompson}@loni.ucla.edu

Abstract. Genetic analysis of diffusion tensor images (DTI) shows great promise in revealing specific genetic variants that affect brain integrity and connectivity. Most genetic studies of DTI analyze voxel-based diffusivity indices in the image space (such as 3D maps of fractional anisotropy) and overlook tract geometry. Here we propose an automated workflow to cluster fibers using a white matter probabilistic atlas and perform genetic analysis on the shape characteristics of fiber tracts. We apply our approach to large study of 4-Tesla high angular resolution diffusion imaging (HARDI) data from 198 healthy, young adult twins (age: 20-30). Illustrative results show heritability for the shapes of several major tracts, as color-coded maps.

Keywords: HARDI, Tractography, Image Registration, White Matter Probabilistic Atlas, Fiber Alignment, Clustering, Curve Matching, Heritability.

1 Introduction

The relationship between genetics, brain structure, and function has long been debated in medicine, sociology, education, and neuroscience. How is the brain influenced by nature (genetics) and nurture (environment)?

Most studies of genetic influences on brain structure use T1-weighted anatomical MRI, which lacks information on white matter fiber tracts in the brain. For two decades, diffusion tensor magnetic resonance imaging (DT-MRI [1]) has been increasingly used to study pathology and connectivity of white matter pathways. DT-MRI provides directional information on water diffusion in brain tissue. Fractional anisotropy (FA), as a measure of microstructural directionality, tends to be higher

---

[*] This study was supported by Grant RO1 HD050735 from the National Institutes of Health (NIH) and Grant 496682 from the National Health and Medical Research Council (NHMRC), Australia.

T. Liu et al. (Eds.): MBIA 2011, LNCS 7012, pp. 35–43, 2011.

when fiber tracts are more directionally coherent. Recent genetic analyses of DT-MRI show moderately high heritability for several diffusivity measures including the FA [2], which is widely considered to be a measure of fiber integrity. Structural equation models and heritability analyses have also been extended to handle the full diffusion tensor [3], and orientation density functions that represent the diffusion process [4]. Significant proportions of the population variability in FA are due to genetic factors. Heritability is detected in several white matter areas, such as the corpus callosum, internal capsule, along others, in voxel-wise FA maps [2].

The major disadvantage of voxel-based analysis of FA is that tract geometry is overlooked. FA maps do not provide information on the geometric characteristics of tract, making it hard to assess genetic effects on their shapes. Brouwer *et al.* [5] assessed genetic and environmental influences on fiber tracts in children by constructing average fiber bundles from manually defined regions of interest; even so, manual seeding of tracts makes it hard to analyze a large dataset, and limits the coverage to a few tracts.

Here we introduce an automated workflow to (1) cluster the results of whole-brain high angular resolution diffusion imaging (HARDI) tractography into anatomically meaningful tracts, and (2) discover genetic contributions to tract shape characteristics, assessing their heritability. It is important to know if a fiber property is heritable; if so, it can be used in the search for specific variants on the genome that contribute to the wiring of the brain. To cluster fibers from whole-brain tractography across a large population, we used a white matter probabilistic atlas, to which all subjects' brain images were non-linearly aligned. Fibers reconstructed from streamline tractography were warped to the same atlas space by applying the deformation fields from the registration step. Clustering was performed based on the probabilistic atlas. Once each tract was extracted, a curve matching method was implemented to find corresponding points on each fiber belonging to that tract across the population. For each tract, shape dispersion measures were analyzed using a statistical model of heritability. A flow chart is shown in **Fig. 1**. We conducted a large population study with this workflow, as detailed next.

2 Methods

2.1 Subjects and Image Acquisition

Participating in this study were 198 healthy young adult twins (mean age: 23.2+/- 2.1SD) from 99 families in Australia. All twins were right-handed. No subjects had any major medical condition or psychiatric illness. All subjects were evaluated to exclude any pathology known to affect brain structure. Diffusion imaging was available in 99 complete pairs – 62 monozygotic pairs (21 male-only pairs) and 37 same-sex dizygotic twin pairs (12 male-only pairs).

Compared to DT-MRI, HARDI [6] allows the use of a complex diffusion model. In fiber tractography, this can allow more accurate reconstruction of fibers that mix and cross, and more sophisticated definitions of diffusion anisotropy when multiple fiber orientations are present in a voxel [7]. HARDI images were acquired with a 4T Bruker Medspec MRI scanner, using single-shot echo planar imaging with parameters: TR/TE = 6090/91.7ms, 23cm FOV, and a 128x128 acquisition matrix.

Each 3D volume consisted of 55 2-mm axial slices, with no gap, and 1.79x1.79mm² in-plane resolution. 105 image volumes were acquired per subject: 11 with no diffusion sensitization, i.e., T2-weighted b_0 images, and 94 diffusion-weighted images ($b = 1159$ s/mm²).

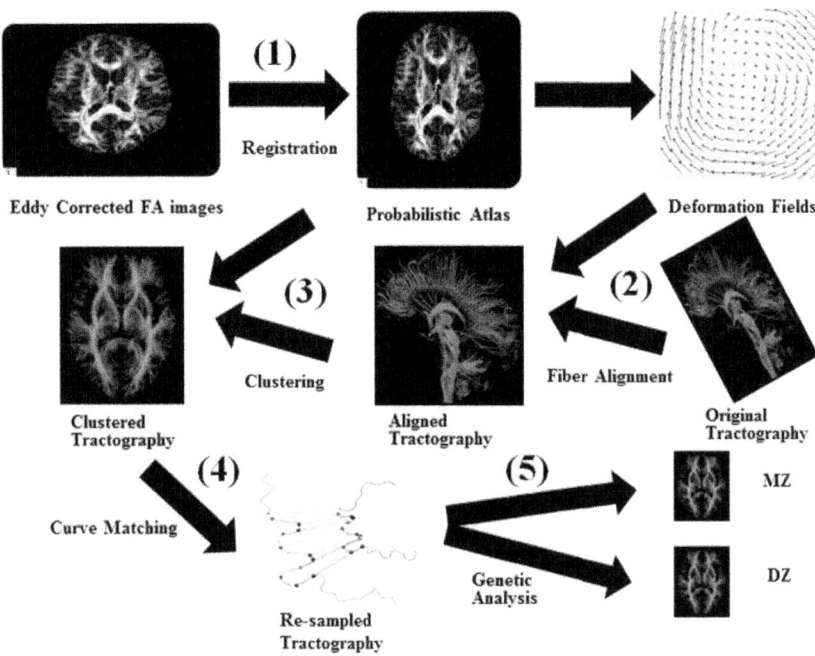

Fig. 1. Flow chart of the image processing steps: (1) Each subject's FA image was nonlinearly registered to the atlas. (2) The resulting deformation fields were applied to the extracted fibers to warp them into the atlas space. (3) Fibers were clustered based on their locations in the atlas. (4) With shaped-based curve matching, we interpolated the points on the fibers corresponding to those on the mean curve of the tract. (5) Genetic analysis was performed on the defined shape metrics.

2.2 Fiber Tractography

The raw HARDI images were corrected for eddy-current induced distortions with FSL [8]. To perform whole-brain tractography, we used the Diffusion Toolkit [9], a software package that uses a streamline algorithm to reconstruct fiber paths. The software applied the Fiber Assignment by Continuous Tracking (FACT)-like method [10] but was based on the HARDI data model that each voxel has multiple principal diffusion directions. We performed whole-brain tractography, with the maximum fiber turning angle set to 35° per voxel.

2.3 Image Registration

Eddy-current corrected diffusion images were skull-stripped using the FSL tool, BET, to facilitate registration. Each subject's fractional anisotropy (FA) map was generated from the 105 diffusion volumes with FSL. Registration was performed on the FA images. The target image was a single-subject FA map in the ICBM-152 space called the "Type II Eve Atlas" [11]. This atlas FA image was 181x217x181, with 1mm isotropic resolution.

Subjects' FA images were first linearly aligned to the atlas with FLIRT in FSL [12], via a 12-parameter affine registration, with mutual information as the cost function, and trilinear interpolation. To improve alignment, all linearly registered FA images were elastically registered to the atlas using inverse-consistent elastic registration [13]. This step used mutual information as a cost function to optimize an elastic deformation using the spectral method (Fast Fourier Transform). The resulting three 64x64x64 resolution deformation fields (x-, y-, and z-direction, respectively) were used to align all subjects' FA images to the atlas coordinate space.

2.4 Fiber Alignment

Fibers generated in **Section 2.2** were aligned to the same coordinate space by applying the affine transformation and deformation fields from the elastic registration in **Section 2.3**. Jin *et al.* [14] previously verified that nonlinear alignment improves analysis of tract data.

2.5 Fiber Clustering

We excluded any fibers with arc lengths <6.5cm, leaving ~15,000 fibers per subject for clustering. This number of fibers was sufficient to represent the cortico-spinal tract and other major white matter structures.

Clustering was based on a spatial probability map of white matter tracts in the atlas, for 47 major tracts [15]. For each fiber in the subject's brain, we matched every point on the fiber to the nearest neighboring voxel to apply information in the probabilistic map. We defined "the fiber probability" of being a particular tract as the mean of the probabilities of the voxels, associated with the corresponding fiber points, which belong to this particular tract in the probabilistic map. Whether a fiber belonged to a particular tract depended on the following 3 criteria: (1) the fiber probability was largest for that particular tract among all tracts; (2) the fiber probability of being this particular tract was at least 0.2; (3) at least 70% of points on the fiber fell into this particular tract.

2.6 Curve Matching

Although many other choices are possible, we used shape dispersion measures to define tract shape. For a given tract, we first calculated the mean curve for the set of fibers in that tract; we then registered all the fibers in the tract to this mean curve;

next, we calculated the mean and standard deviation of the distances from the corresponding points on each fiber inside this tract to those on the mean curve.

To compute each tract's average shape, we used a representation proposed in Joshi *et al.* [16][17]. This representation used a square-root velocity function to represent open curves. Given a unit-length curve $\beta: [0,1] \rightarrow R^3$, its shape is represented by a function $q: [0,1] \rightarrow R^3$ such that $q = \dot{\beta}/\sqrt{|\dot{\beta}|}$, where $\dot{\beta}$ represents the derivative of β. Therefore, a fiber curve in the native space is transported to its shape in the space of all q functions that assume this square-root velocity form. An important ingredient for computing the mean shape is the establishment of geodesics between shapes. A geodesic is a shortest path between two points in a space. The mean curve for a fiber tract is the one minimizing the sum of the squared pairwise geodesic distances to all individual fibers of that bundle.

To compute corresponding points across the subjects, first, for any individual tract, a mean curve based on the sampled points was calculated for each subject; then, a population mean curve was generated with the information on those individual mean curves for each subject; in turn, the parameterization of the population mean curve was projected back onto the individual mean curve; finally, every fiber that belonged to this tract for each subject was re-sampled, based on the re-sampled individual mean curve.

2.7 Genetic Analysis

Monozygotic (MZ) twins share 100% of their genetic variants whereas dizygotic (DZ) twins share, on average 50%, of their genes. A simple and widely-used estimate of heritability, in twin studies, assesses how much the intra-class correlation for MZ twin pairs (r_{MZ}) exceeds the DZ twin correlation (r_{DZ}). Falconer's heritability statistic [18] is defined as $h^2 = 2(r_{MZ} - r_{DZ})$. It estimates the proportion of the overall variance that is due to genetic differences among individuals. Here, the measures we chose in **Section 2.6** (the mean and the standard deviation of the distances from the points on each fiber to the corresponding points on the mean curve) were used to calculate intra-class correlations r_{MZ} and r_{DZ}. When $h^2 = 0$, there is no evidence of a genetic effect; $h^2 = 1$ implies all of the variance is due to genetic factors.

3 Results

3.1 Clustering

Fig. 2 shows clustering results (*top, front, and side views*) in a representative subject. Major tracts, distinguished in color, include the cortico-spinal tracts, thalamo-cortical tracts to primary motor and frontal areas, multiple sectors of the corpus callosum, the cingulum, and the superior and inferior longitudinal fasciculi.

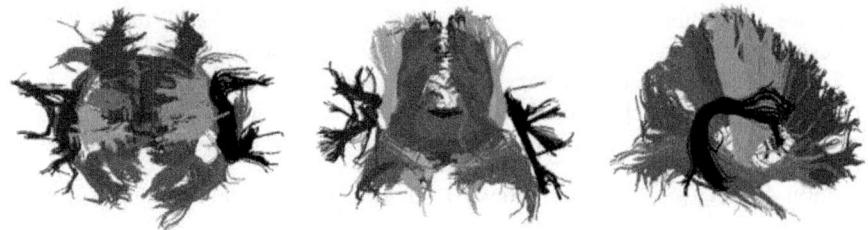

Fig. 2. A representative clustering result for 4-Tesla 105-gradient HARDI data from one individual subject, showing major white matter tracts. Top, front, and side views are shown.

Fig. 3 shows clustering results for several tracts in four different subjects (no twin pairs). Despite some individual variations, the overall tract shapes are consistent across the population. The tracts are the left cortico-spinal tract (inferior-superior orientation) in *yellow*, the callosal *genu* (left-right orientation) in *red*, and the left cingulum (posterior-anterior orientation) in *green*.

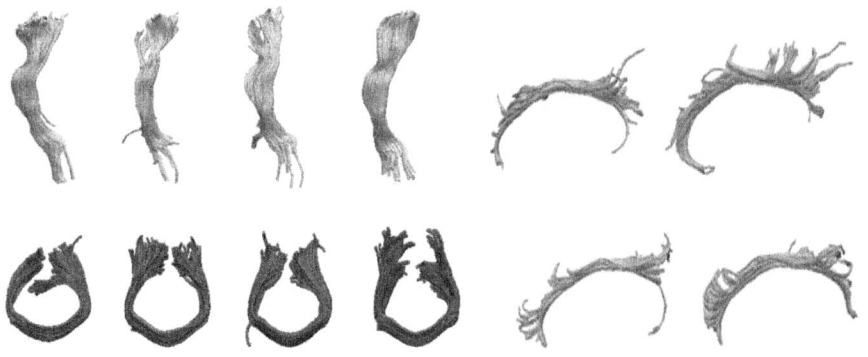

Fig. 3. The left cortico-spinal tracts for 4 different subjects (not members of the same twin pair) are shown in *yellow*. The tract running through the callosal *genu* is shown in *red*, and the left cingulum tract is shown in *green*.

3.2 Genetic Analyses

Fig. 4 shows color maps of Falconer's heritability statistic, based on the mean and the standard deviation of distances between individual fibers and the mean curve for a particular tract (as in **Section 2.6**). The mean distance is related to the thickness of a tract. The left panel of each figure shows the mean and the right panel shows the standard deviation. **Fig. 4(a), 4(b), and 4(c)** show the left corti-cospinal tract, the callosal *genu,* and the left cingulum bundle.

In **Fig. 4(a)**, greater heritability is detected near the cortex, perhaps because the overall variability across subjects is greater there. Minimal genetic influence is detected for the mean distances in the callosal *genu* in **Fig. 4(b)**, but there is some influence on the standard deviation of distances. An opposite trend is found for the

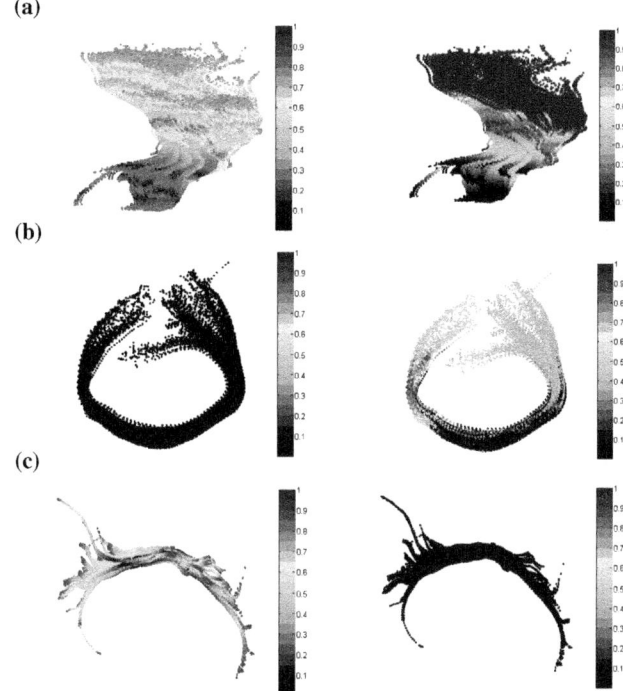

Fig. 4. Color maps show Falconer's heritability statistic for **(a)** the mean distances (*left*) and the standard deviations of distances (*right*) of the left corticospinal tract; **(b)** the mean distances (*left*) and the standard deviations of distances (*right*) of the tract that runs through the callosal *genu*; **(c)** the mean distances (*left*) and the standard deviations of distances (*right*) of the left cingulum tract.

left cingulum tract in **Fig. 4(c)**. These maps are exploratory, and the patterns will be verifiable when larger cohorts of subjects are available.

4   Conclusion

Here we proposed an automated framework for genetic analysis of clustered fiber tracts in a large population. We focused on geometric properties of the tracts, such as their local thickness (which is related to the mean distance of fibers to a central curve), and their dispersion. These features were heritable, and therefore may offer promising targets to screen for specific genetic polymorphisms that influence tract geometry.

As this was a large, multi-subject study, nonlinear registration of HARDI was used to better align fibers prior to atlas-based clustering. We have found that atlas based clustering can give more anatomically interpretable tracts than spectral approaches that use geometric information about the fibers themselves, but combining both types of information may offer additional benefits in the future.

The tract shape measures we defined are basic, intuitive parameters that may not fully represent the characteristics of tract geometry. More sophisticated measures will be defined, in future, to more fully characterize tract shapes, and how they interrelate. In addition, as the sample size increases, we will fit more complex structural equation models to separate genetic (A), shared environmental (C), and unique environmental (E) components of the variance.

This is a high-throughput workflow, and avoids the inefficiency of manually seeded approaches. It may expedite the discovery and replication of specific genetic polymorphisms associated with tract characteristics.

References

1. Basser, P.J., et al.: MR Diffusion Tensor Spectroscopy and Imaging. Biophys. J. 66, 259–267 (1994)
2. Chiang, M.C., et al.: Genetics of White Matter Development: A DTI Study of 705 Twins and Their Siblings Aged 12 to 29. NeuroImage 54, 2308–2317 (2011)
3. Lee, A.D., et al.: Multivariate Variance-Components Analysis in DTI. In: The 2010 IEEE International Symposium on Biomedical Imaging (ISBI): from Nano to Macro, pp. 1157–1160. IEEE Press, Piscataway (2010)
4. Lepore, N., et al.: A Multivariate Groupwise Genetic Analysis of White Matter Integrity using Orientation Distribution Functions. In: The 2010 Medical Image Computing and Computer Assisted Intervention (MICCAI) Workshop on Computational Diffusion MRI (CDMRI), Beijing, China, pp. 1–11 (2010)
5. Brouwer, R.M., et al.: Heritability of DTI and MTR in Nine-year-old Children. NeuroImage 53, 1085–1092 (2010)
6. Tuch, D.S.: Q-Ball Imaging. Magn. Reson. Med. 52, 1358–1372 (2004)
7. Leow, A.D., et al.: The Tensor Distribution Function. Magn. Reson. Med. 61, 205–214 (2009)
8. FSL, http://www.fmrib.ox.ac.uk/fsl/
9. Diffusion Toolkit, http://trackvis.org/dtk/
10. Mori, S., et al.: Three-dimensional Tracking of Axonal Projections in the Brain by Magnetic Resonance Imaging. Ann. Neurol. 45, 265–269 (1999)
11. Oishi, K., et al.: Atlas-based Whole Brain White Matter Analysis using Large Deformation Diffeomorphic Metric Mapping: Application to Normal Elderly and Alzheimer's Disease Participants. NeuroImage 46, 486–499 (2009)
12. Jenkinson, M., Smith, S.M.: A Global Optimisation Method for Robust Affine Registration of Brain Images. Medical Image Analysis 5, 143–156 (2001)
13. Leow, A.D., et al.: Statistical Properties of Jacobian Maps and the Realization of Unbiased Large-deformation Nonlinear Image Registration. IEEE Trans. Med. Imaging 26, 822–832 (2007)
14. Jin, Y., et al.: 3D Elastic Registration Improves HARDI-derived Fiber Alignment and Automated Tract Clustering. In: The 2011 IEEE International Symposium on Biomedical Imaging (ISBI): from Nano to Macro, pp. 822–826. IEEE Press, Piscataway (2011)
15. Zhang, Y., et al.: Atlas-Guided Tract Reconstruction for Automated and Comprehensive Examination of the White Matter Anatomy. NeuroImage 52, 1289–1301 (2010)

16. Joshi, S.H., et al.: Removing Shape-Preserving Transformations in Square-Root Elastic (SRE) Framework for Shape Analysis of Curves. In: Yuille, A.L., Zhu, S.-C., Cremers, D., Wang, Y. (eds.) EMMCVPR 2007. LNCS, vol. 4679, pp. 387–398. Springer, Heidelberg (2007)
17. Joshi, S.H., et al.: A Novel Representation for Riemannian Analysis of Elastic Curves in R^n. In: IEEE Conference on Computer Vision and Pattern Recognition (CVPR), Minneapolis, Minnesota, USA, pp. 1–7 (2007)
18. Falconer, D., Mackay, T.F.: Introduction to Quantitative Genetics, 4th edn. Benjamin Cummings (1996)

Ordinal Ranking for Detecting Mild Cognitive Impairment and Alzheimer's Disease Based on Multimodal Neuroimages and CSF Biomarkers

Yong Fan and The Alzheimer's Disease Neuroimaging Initiative (ADNI)[*]

National Laboratory of Pattern Recognition, Institute of Automation
Chinese Academy of Sciences, Beijing, 100190, China
yong.fan@ieee.org, yfan@nlpr.ia.ac.cn

Abstract. Early diagnosis of Alzheimer's disease (AD) based on neuroimaging and fluid biomarker data has attracted a lot of interest in medical image analysis. Most existing studies have been focusing on two-class classification problems, e.g., distinguishing AD patients from cognitive normal (CN) elderly or distinguishing mild cognitive impairment (MCI) individuals from CN elderly. However, to achieve the goal of early diagnosis of AD, we need to identify individuals with AD and MCI, especially MCI individuals who will convert to AD, in a single setting, which essentially is a multi-class classification problem. In this paper, we propose an ordinal ranking based classification method for distinguishing CN, MCI non-converter (MCI-NC), MCI converter (MCI-C), and AD at an individual level, taking into account the inherent ordinal severity of brain damage caused by normal aging, MCI, and AD, rather than formulating the classification as a multi-class classification problem. Experiment results indicate that the proposed method can achieve a better performance than traditional multi-class classification techniques based on multimodal neuroimaging and CSF biomarker data of the ADNI.

Keywords: Ordinal ranking, Alzheimer's disease, Mild cognitive impairment, MCI converters, Neuroimaging, Fluid biomarker.

1   Introduction

AD is the most common dementia and its current clinical diagnosis is based on neuropsychological and neurobehavioral examinations which have so much variability. Therefore there is an urgent need for biomarkers that are both sensitive and specific for early and improved diagnosis. Since AD related degenerative histological changes occur long before the disease is clinically detectable, there has been a keen interest to develop imaging-based biomarkers.

Neuroimaging techniques, including structural MRI, PET, and other imaging modalities, have been investigated as surrogate markers of AD pathology. Structural MRI has shown that AD pathology is associated with medial temporal lobe atrophy, especially of the hippocampus (HIP) and the entorhinal cortex (EC) [1]. PET imaging

---

[*] Data used in the preparation of this article were obtained from the ADNI database.

T. Liu et al. (Eds.): MBIA 2011, LNCS 7012, pp. 44–51, 2011.
© Springer-Verlag Berlin Heidelberg 2011

has demonstrated that abnormal glucose metabolism and amyloid load in brains of MCI and AD patients may be quantified at brain regions, such as HIP, inferior parietal lobe, middle frontal gyrus, and posterior cingulate cortex [2]. However, the pattern of AD pathology is complex and evolves as the disease progresses [3]. Therefore, measuring regional volumes or glucose metabolism at a few brain regions cannot capture the spatiotemporal pattern of AD pathology in its entirety.

AD's pathology is characterized by the presence of amyloid plaques and neurofibrillary tangles in the brain. Lots of effort has been made to measure the amyloid and tangle proteins in the brain indirectly from blood and CSF, especially the latter due to its direct contact with the brain. Although not highly specific, CSF measures of amyloid-beta and tau have been demonstrated sensitive to AD [4, 5]. Specifically, AD is often associated with elevated concentration of tau and decreased level of amyloid-beta.

Since fluid biomarkers and neuroimaging data provide complementary information about the brain, effort has been made to improve the biomarkers' performance by combining neuroimaging and CSF biomarkers [1, 6]. These studies, combining CSF biomarkers with either structural MRI or functional imaging, all demonstrated that the combination of complementary information can potentially improve the diagnosis performance of AD.

Techniques of multivariate pattern classification have been increasingly adopted in neuroimaging studies of AD [7-11], aiming to provide tools that classify individuals, based on their MRI and/or PET scans, rather than determining statistical group differences. The multivariate pattern classification methods, optimally combining information of multiple measures derived from images, have demonstrated that the classification of individuals can be achieved with relatively high classification accuracy in a variety of neuroimaging studies [7-13]. Recent studies have also shown that the combination of neuroimaging and CSF biomarker measures can improve the classification performance of AD [14]. Most existing classification studies of AD have been focusing on two-class classification problems, e.g., distinguishing AD patients from CN elderly. However, the early diagnosis of AD is essentially a multi-class classification problem, i.e., we need to identify individuals with AD, MCI-C, and MCI-NC in a single setting.

The multi-class classification problem associated with early diagnosis of AD can be solved in a typical multi-class classification framework, using strategies of one-against-one or one-against-the rest [15]. However, such typical multi-class classification methods may overlook ordinal information of the damage rendered by normal aging, MCI and AD. To make the best of inherent ordinal severity of brain damage at AD's different stages, we propose an ordinal ranking method to distinguish AD, MCI-C, and MCI-NC from CN based on multimodal neuroimaging and CSF biomarker data.

2   Methods

2.1   Ordinal Ranking for Classification of CN, MCI-NC, MCI-C, and AD

Early diagnosis of AD requires not only the classification of CN, MCI, and AD, but also the identification of MCI converters. As a transitional state from CN to AD, MCI might correspond to several different degrees of brain damage, as reflected by the fact that individuals with MCI may convert to AD at an annual rate as high as 15%, and some MCI individuals do not convert to AD even ten years after the onset of memory problems [16]. Roughly speaking, brain change rendered by normal aging, MCI-NC, MCI-C, and AD comes with an increased severity of brain damage that is ranked, but difficult to be assigned with a metric value. The inter-subject variability might obliterate the relatively small differences between CN and MCI-NC, between MCI-NC and MCI-C, as well as between MCI-C and AD, which makes a difficult task for discriminating different stages of AD progression. Since no proper metric distance can be defined for the ordinal damage severity, metric regression methods might be not good for the problem too.

To make the best of the ordinal severity of the brain damage rendered by normal aging, MCI, and AD, we propose an ordinal ranking method within an ordinal regression framework by transferring the ordinal ranking problem into a set of binary "larger than" problems [17, 18].

For our problem, CN, MCI-NC, MCI-C, and AD are labeled using an ordinal order $y \in \{1,2,3,4\}$, corresponding to their severity of brain damage. Three binary "larger than" problems associated with the ordinal ranking problem are damage "larger than normal aging?" ($y > 1$), "larger than MCI-NC?" ($y > 2$), and "larger than MCI-C?" ($y > 3$). Particularly, the binary "larger than" classification problems are solved separately in a cost sensitive learning framework so that flexible binary classifiers with distinctive features can be constructed to best fit different sub-problems [18].

Given training data $\{(x_i, y_i), i = 1, \dots, n\}$, where x_i is a feature vector and its associated label is $y_i \in \{1,2,3,4\}$, for each particular binary problem $(y > k)$, its positively labeled training dataset X_k^+ and negatively labeled training dataset X_k^- are constructed as following [18]:

$$X_k^+ = \{(x_i, 1)|y_i > k\}, \ X_k^- = \{(x_i, -1)|y_i \leq k\}. \tag{1}$$

Obviously, for each particular binary classification problem, the cost of miss classification of different samples is not equal. For example, in the "larger than normal aging" problem, the miss classification of AD samples is associated with larger cost than the miss classification of MCI-NC samples, whereas in the "larger than MCI-C" problem, the miss classification of CN samples is associated with larger cost than the miss classification of MCI-NC samples. Taking the cost associated with miss classification into account, for a binary classification problem $(y > k)$, we use a cost coding scheme for samples with label y, defined as:

$$\text{Cost}_k(y) = \exp(\alpha|y - k - 0.5|), \tag{2}$$

where α is a parameter to weight the miss classification cost for different samples.

To solve the cost sensitive binary classification problem $(y > k)$, a weighed SVM method is adopted [19] to minimize the cost sensitive classification error:

$$\min_{w_k, b_k, \xi} \frac{1}{2} w_k^T w_k + C \sum_i \text{Cost}_k(y_i) \xi_i \tag{3}$$

Subject to $z_k(y_i)(w_k^T \phi_k(x_i)w_k + b_k) \geq 1 - \xi_i, \ \xi_i \geq 0, i = 1, \dots, n,$

where $z_k(y_i) = 1$, if $y_i > k$, otherwise $z_k(y_i) = -1$, ϕ_k is an implicit mapping function associated with the kernel function $K_k(x_i, x_j) = \phi_k(x_i)^T \phi_k(x_j)$, and (w_k, b_k) are parameters of the SVM decision function f_k.

Once all the binary classifiers are constructed, an ordinal ranking rule is constructed as [17, 18]:

$$r(x) = 1 + \sum_{k=1}^{3} [\![f_k(x) > 0]\!], \tag{4}$$

where $[\![\cdot]\!]$ is 1 if the inner condition is true, and 0 otherwise.

2.2   Feature Extraction and Selection

Feature extraction

The classification system is built on measures computed from imaging and fluid biomarkers provided by the ADNI project. For CSF biomarker, three measures are available, including $A\beta_{1-42}$, t-tau and p-tau. These CSF biomarker measures are directly used in the ordinal classification.

The imaging data provided by the ADNI project consist of structure MRI and FDG-PET scans, from which regional brain volume measures and regional PET values are computed using atlas warping. Particularly, geometric distortion corrected MR images are used, and PET images are co-registered with their associated MR images. The MR images are segmented using new segmentation tool and further deformed to a custom brain template generated from 100 MR images of CN subjects without PET scans using DARTEL [20]. The PET images are also deformed to the template space using their corresponding MR images' deformation fields. Finally, AAL template is used to partition the brain template space into regions of interest (ROI) [21]. The gray matter volume of each ROI is calculated for each subject by summing its corresponding modulated gray matter tissue density values. The PET value of each ROI is calculated for each subject by averaging its PET intensities and normalized using the PET value of cerebellum. The normalized gray matter volume and PET value measures of cortical and subcortical ROIs are used as features in the ordinal classification.

Feature selection

From imaging and fluid biomarker data, many measures can be computed as features for classification, however not all of them are informative for classification.

To find the discriminative features, a ranking based feature selection technique is adopted. In particular, Spearman's rho is used to rank features based on training data, taking the ordinal information of samples' labels into account, although other measures can be similarly adopted here. To make the feature ranking robust to outliers, a leave-one-out procedure is used to compute the Spearman's rho and a conservative principle is applied to select the minimal absolute Spearman's rho for gauging each feature's discriminative power [13]. The top ranked features are to be used to build SVM classifiers. In our problem, the most discriminative feature sets might be distinctive for different binary "larger than" problems.

2.3   Parameter Optimization and Bagging Classification

The parameters of the classification system, e.g., SVM's trade-off parameter C and the number of top ranked features used in classification, have to be estimated by cross-validation. However, it can inevitably decrease the classification power if we separate the limited training samples into small training and validation datasets for parameter tuning. Furthermore, the individual variability of brain anatomy, function, and measures derived from fluid biomarkers may render the classification less stable if small changes in the training set result in large changes in predictions.

To improve the stability of classification, as well as to facilitate automatic parameter selection without decreasing the statistical power, we use a bagging strategy to build ensemble classifiers [7, 22]. Within this framework, for each binary "larger than" classification problem, rather than building a single classifier, we build an ensemble of classifiers, with base classifiers built using SVM with top ranked features. Such strategy has been demonstrated to be successful in brain image classification studies [7]. First, replications of the training samples are generated based on a k-fold random sampling strategy. Second, base classifiers are built upon the replications of training samples. The parameters involved in the algorithm are to be determined by optimizing the performance of the trained base classifiers on the left-out training samples (excluded from the current training subset). Finally, once the base classifiers are built based on different training subsets, an ensemble classifier is constructed by combining their outputs on test samples using voting.

3   Experiment Results

We tested our approach on an ADNI dataset, consisting of 207 subjects, each of them having baseline structural MR image, FDG-PET scan, and CSF biomarker data. The demographic and clinical details of these subjects are shown in Table 1.

Table 1. Demographic and clinical details of the subjects at the time of baseline data collection. The average time that elapsed between the baseline scans and conversion of MCI-C to AD was 23.3 ±12.0 (mean ± std) months.

	CN (n=55)	MCI-NC (n=57)	MCI-C (n=44)	AD (n=51)
Gender(male)	36	41	27	33
Age(year)	75.1±5.0	74.5±7.1	75.5±7.2	75.4±7.6
Edu (year)	15.8±3.1	16.0±3.0	15.9±2.8	14.8±3.7
MMSE	29.0±1.2	27.4±1.5	26.7±1.8	23.8±1.9

A 10-fold cross-validation procedure was adopted to evaluate the performance of our approach. In each fold, a 5-fold based bagging ranker was constructed. In particular, linear SVMs were used to build binary classifiers, therefore the parameters to be estimated were the number of top ranked features, SVM's trade-off parameter C, and the parameter α for tuning the miss classification cost. These parameters were optimized using the method described in section 2.3. For comparison purpose, using the same cross-validation procedure, a one-against-one based multi-class classification was applied to the same dataset too. For each one-against-one classification, an aggregated binary classifier was constructed using the same feature ranking and parameter optimization strategy. The classification results are summarized in Table 2 for our proposed approach and the traditional multi-class classification enhanced by feature selection.

Table 2. Ten-fold cross-validation results of ordinal ranking (left) and multi-class classification (right). Each row of the table shows the numbers of testing subjects of different states are classified as CN, MCI-NC, MCI-C, and AD.

ordinal	CN	MCI-NC	MCI-C	AD
CN	27	18	8	2
MCI-NC	9	23	19	6
MCI-C	4	17	17	6
AD	1	8	28	14

multi-class	CN	MCI-NC	MCI-C	AD
CN	36	15	4	0
MCI-NC	20	18	12	7
MCI-C	7	16	8	13
AD	3	19	11	18

As shown in Table 2, our proposed approach achieved a better performance than the traditional multi-class classification method enhanced by feature selection. Although the classification performance was not good enough to be used in clinic practice, our approach demonstrated a very good trend to achieve an acceptable accuracy, observing that 1) 9% MCI-C subjects was classified as CN, and 2) only 2% AD subjects were classified as CN. The classification results of MCI subjects also reflect the fact that early diagnosis of MCI-C is more difficult [9, 23].

The binary classifiers constituting the ordinal ranking rule were built on the top ranked imaging and CSF biomarker measures. It has been observed that the CSF measures were selected in almost all the binary classification problems. The contribution of imaging features to the classification is visualized by overlapping ROIs whose imaging features were selected with higher frequency in the classification. As shown in Fig. 1, the imaging measures were mainly from brain regions that have been demonstrated to be affected by AD in many existing AD studies, e.g., cortical regions of temporal lobe. The increased spatial complexity of imaging pattern associated with the binary "larger than" problems also reflects the ordinal severity of brain damage of AD.

4   Discussion and Conclusions

We have presented an ordinal ranking method for classifying AD's different stages using multimodal neuroimaging and CSF biomarker data. The comparison with the traditional multi-class classification methods shows that our method can achieve a promising performance, indicating that the utilization of inherent ordinal severity of brain damage rendered by AD's different stages can help achieve improved classification performance. The current implementation of our method utilized relatively simple imaging features, i.e., ROI gray matter volumes and PET values. The performance of our method might be further improved if the correlation between different modalities is taken into account [7] and advanced feature extraction techniques, e.g., adaptive regional feature extraction [13], are used. Besides

Classifier
(y>1)
"larger than
normal
aging?"

Classifier
(y>2)
"larger than
MCI-NC?"

Classifier
(y>3)
"larger than
MCI-C?"

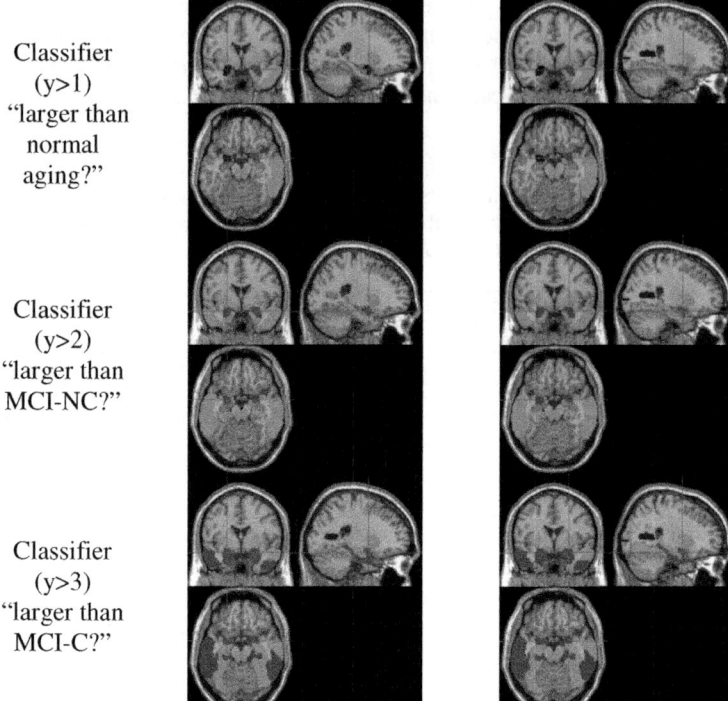

Fig. 1. Brain regions selected with higher frequency in different binary "larger than" problems. ROIs in blue color indicate that their gray matter volume measures contributed to the classification, ROIs in green color indicate that their PET value measures contributed to the classification, and ROIs in red color indicate that both gray matter volume and PET value measures contributed to the classification.

classification, our proposed method is also a better fit for regression studies of AD associated clinical score estimation than metric regression [24, 25], since most of the clinical score measures, e.g., mini mental state examination (MMSE), are not continuous variables too.

Acknowledgements. This study was partially supported by the National Science Foundation of China (No. 30970770) and the Hundred Talents Program of the Chinese Academy of Sciences.

References

1. de Leon, M.J., et al.: Imaging and CSF Studies in the Preclinical Diagnosis of Alzheimer's Disease. Annals of the New York Academy of Sciences 1097, 114–145 (2007)
2. Li, Y., et al.: Regional analysis of FDG and PIB-PET images in normal aging, mild cognitive impairment, and Alzheimer's disease. European Journal of Nuclear Medicine and Molecular Imaging 35, 2169–2181 (2008)
3. Braak, H., et al.: Evolution of Alzheimer's disease related cortical lesions. Journal of Neural Transmission Supplementum 54, 97–106 (1998)

4. Parnetti, L., et al.: Diagnosing prodromal Alzheimer's disease: Role of CSF biochemical markers. Mechanisms of Ageing and Development 127, 129–132 (2006)
5. Shaw, L.M., et al.: Cerebrospinal fluid biomarker signature in Alzheimer's disease neuroimaging initiative subjects. Annals of Neurology 65, 403–413 (2009)
6. de Leon, M., et al.: Longitudinal CSF and MRI biomarkers improve the diagnosis of mild cognitive impairment. Neurobiology of Aging 27, 394–401 (2006)
7. Fan, Y., et al.: Structural and functional biomarkers of prodromal Alzheimer's disease: A high-dimensional pattern classification study. NeuroImage 41, 277–285 (2008)
8. Davatzikos, C., et al.: Detection of prodromal Alzheimer's disease via pattern classification of magnetic resonance imaging. Neurobiology of Aging 29, 514–523 (2008)
9. Fan, Y., et al.: Spatial patterns of brain atrophy in MCI patients, identified via high-dimensional pattern classification, predict subsequent cognitive decline. Neuroimage 39, 1731–1743 (2008)
10. Kloppel, S., et al.: Automatic classification of MR scans in Alzheimer's disease. Brain 131, 681–689 (2008)
11. Vemuri, P., et al.: Alzheimer's disease diagnosis in individual subjects using structural MR images: Validation studies. Neuroimage 39, 1186–1197 (2008)
12. Fan, Y., et al.: Unaffected Family Members and Schizophrenia Patients Share Brain Structure Patterns: a High-Dimensional Pattern Classification Study Biological Psychiatry. Biological Psychiatry 63, 118–124 (2008)
13. Fan, Y., et al.: COMPARE: Classification Of Morphological Patterns using Adaptive Regional Elements. IEEE Transactions on Medical Imaging 26, 93–105 (2007)
14. Zhang, D.Q., et al.: Multimodal classification of Alzheimer's disease and mild cognitive impairment. NeuroImage 55, 856–867 (2011)
15. Hsu, C.-W., et al.: A comparison of methods for multi-class support vector machines. IEEE Transactions on Neural Networks 13, 415–425 (2002)
16. Petersen, R.C.: Mild cognitive impairment: Aging to Alzheimer's Disease. Oxford University Press, Oxford (2003)
17. Li, L., et al.: Ordinal Regression by Extended Binary Classification. Advances in Neural Information Processing Systems 19, 865–872 (2007)
18. Chang, K.-Y., et al.: Ordinal Hyperplanes Ranker with Cost Sensitivities for Age Estimation. In: IEEE Conference on Computer Vision and Pattern Recognition (CVPR), Colorado (Springs 2011)
19. Chang, C.-C., et al.: LIBSVM: A library for support vector machines. ACM Transactions on Intelligent Systems and Technology 2, 27:21–27:27 (2011)
20. Ashburner, J.: A fast diffeomorphic image registration algorithm. NeuroImage 38, 95–113 (2007)
21. Tzourio-Mazoyer, N., et al.: Automated Anatomical Labeling of Activations in SPM Using a Macroscopic Anatomical Parcellation of the MNI MRI Single-Subject Brain. NeuroImage 15, 273–289 (2002)
22. Breiman, L.: Bagging predictors. Machine Learning 24, 123–140 (1996)
23. Misra, C., et al.: Baseline and longitudinal patterns of brain atrophy in MCI patients, and their use in prediction of short-term conversion to AD: Results from ADNI. NeuroImage 44, 1415–1422 (2009)
24. Wang, Y., et al.: High-dimensional pattern regression using machine learning: From medical images to continuous clinical variables. NeuroImage 50, 1519–1535
25. Fan, Y., et al.: Joint estimation of multiple clinical variables of neurological diseases from imaging patterns. In: Proceedings of the 2010 IEEE international conference on Biomedical Imaging: from Nano to Macro. IEEE Press, Rotterdam (2010)

Manual Annotation, 3-D Shape Reconstruction, and Traumatic Brain Injury Analysis

Lyubomir Zagorchev[1,3], Ardeshir Goshtasby[2], Keith Paulsen[3],
Thomas McAllister[3], Stewart Young[4], and Juergen Weese[4]

[1] Philips Research North America, Briarcliff Manor, NY 10510, USA
[2] Wright State University, Dayton, OH 45435, USA
[3] Dartmouth College, Hanover, NH 03755, USA
[4] Philips Research Hamburg, Hamburg D-22335, Germany
lyubomir.zagorchev@philips.com

Abstract. Bitmask drawing is still the established standard for manual annotation of brain structures by experts. To alleviate problems such as bitmask inconsistencies between slices that lead to jagged contours in corresponding orthogonal cross-sections, we propose a 2-D spline-based contour editing tool in combination with a new algorithm for surface reconstruction from 3-D point clouds. This approach uses a new implicit surface formulation that adapts to the local density of points. We show that manual segmentation of the brainstem, cerebellum, corpus callosum, caudate, putamen, hippocampus and thalamus can be performed with high reproducibility in Magnetic Resonance (MR) data and sufficient accuracy to analyze volume changes for mild Traumatic Brain Injury (TBI) patients. In addition, we show that the new surface reconstruction method allows to reconstruct the shape of brain structures such as the brainstem better than other established surface reconstruction approaches. Our tool can, therefore, not only be used for volume measurements, but may also be used to assess local shape changes of brain structures going along with the progression of neuro-degenerative diseases such as TBI.

Keywords: neuro segmentation, manual tracing, surface recovery.

1 Introduction

Interactive user-controlled bitmap tracing of boundaries has been the established standard for generating brain structure annotations in high-resolution neuro MR images for many years [1]. On the one hand, these annotations are required for clinical studies that quantitatively analyze brain structures and its relation to diseases such as TBI or Alzheimer's [1,6]. On the other hand, these annotations are essential for the development, training and validation of semi- and fully-automatic segmentation techniques [2,9].

Current tools (e.g Slicer, ITK-Snap) for expert neuro-segmentation provide a user interface for manual drawing of bitmasks over the image grid, as illustrated in Figure 1. However, those widely used applications suffer a number of

T. Liu et al. (Eds.): MBIA 2011, LNCS 7012, pp. 52–59, 2011.
© Springer-Verlag Berlin Heidelberg 2011

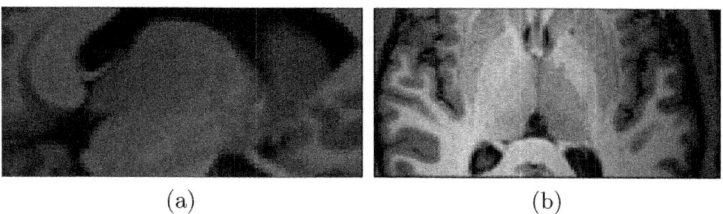

(a) (b)

Fig. 1. Problems associated with the manual bitmask drawing: (a) digitization of a traced structure, and (b) uneven boundaries in orthogonal cross-sections

limitations. First, the obtained 3-D bitmasks are, by definition, constrained to the sampling rate of the image. The smoothness of the resulting segmentation depends on the resolution of the volume as defined by its voxel size. That could lead to large inaccuracies, especially in cases where experts have to segment very small brain structures. In addition, the voxel size digitizes the drawing grid and makes the segmentation, and subsequent correction, of adjacent structures very difficult. Furthermore, while the segmentation may look smooth in the segmentation plane (as seen in Figure 1(a)), it is usually very uneven and jagged in corresponding orthogonal cross-sections (as seen in Figure 1(b)). That effect forces tracers to repeat the manual segmentation in each orthogonal direction, which triples the amount of effort. To alleviate the problems associated with the bitmask drawing, we developed a 2-D spline-based contour editing tool allowing to annotate images with sub-voxel accuracy. The manually defined contours are used to generate a 3-D point cloud representation for each traced structure. A new algorithm for surface reconstruction was developed and applied to the point clouds. The algorithm uses an implicit surface formulation with very narrow basis functions where density of points is high, and very wide basis functions where the density of points is low. The tool has been used by clinicians to annotate the brainstem, cerebellum, corpus callosum, caudate, putamen, hippocampus and thalamus in high resolution neuro MR images of 16 mild TBI patients and 26 healthy volunteers. We present and discuss the result quantitatively for brain volume measurements and show qualitatively that the new surface reconstruction method allows to reconstruct the shape of brain structures such as the brainstem better than other established surface reconstruction approaches.

2   Methods

Volumetric brain structures can be defined using parametric spline contours represented in the continuous space of the volume, as opposed to the image grid. The advantages of that approach over manual bitmask drawing include a sub-voxel resolution, local control and ease of editing, and exact analytical representation. As illustrated in Figure 2(a) and (b), spline contours are not constrained by the spatial resolution of the volume. In addition, the interactive manipulation of control points allows the user to modify/edit only a number of local spline segments while the rest of the curve remains unchanged. A 3-D point cloud representation of a traced structure can be obtained by sampling all of its parameterized planer contours. Please note that the spline contours can be sampled at an arbitrary resolution in the tracing plane. Furthermore, corresponding spline points on different contours can be linearly interpolated. That allows for generation of point clouds with different resolution and density of points from the same set of spline contours, as illustrated in Figure 2 (c) and (d). In fact, resolution much higher than the voxel size of the volume can be accomplished. As a result, the boundary surface of the traced structure can be determined by surface fitting of the 3-D point cloud.

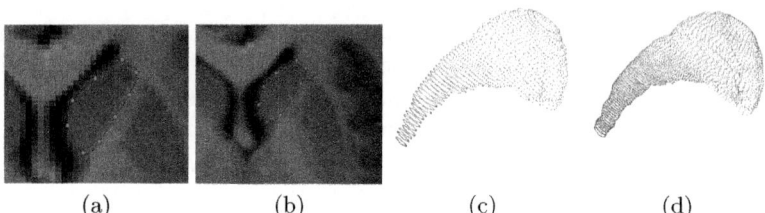

| (a) | (b) | (c) | (d) |

Fig. 2. Advantages of using spline contours include: (a) sub-voxel resolution, (b) better visualization by interpolating texture, and (c) and (d) different point cloud resolutions.

A new method that has the ability to fit a smooth surface to a set of arbitrarily distributed points in 3-D by automatically adjusting the surface parameters to the local density and distribution of the points was developed specifically for this work. Given a set of irregularly spaced points in 3-D,

$$\{\mathbf{p}_i = (x_i, y_i, z_i) : i = 1, \dots, N\}, \tag{1}$$

an implicit surface can be defined as the zero-crossings of the sum of anisotropic signed fields centered at the points. First, let us consider centering an isotropic 3-D Gaussian field at each point and adding the fields together:

$$f_1(x, y, z) = \sum_{i=1}^{N} G_i(\sigma, x, y, z), \tag{2}$$

where $G_i(\sigma, x, y, z)$ is a 3-D Gaussian of magnitude 1 and standard deviation σ centered at point (x_i, y_i, z_i). Rather than centering the same Gaussian at every point, the standard deviation of the Gaussian at a point can be set proportional to the average distance of a fixed number of closest neighbors:

$$f_2(x, y, z) = \sum_{i=1}^{N} G_i(\sigma_i, x, y, z). \tag{3}$$

When isotropic Gaussian fields are centered at the points, local smoothing will be performed equally in all directions. To preserve surface details while reducing noise, it is required to smooth points in flat areas more than in curved areas of a surface. Therefore, a 3-D Gaussian is replaced by three 1-D Gaussians:

$$G_i(\sigma_i, X, Y, Z) = G_i(\sigma_i, X)G_i(\sigma_i, Y)G_i(\sigma_i, Z), \tag{4}$$

where X, Y, and Z represent the local coordinate system of the ith point, with Z pointing in the direction of surface normal and XY showing the tangent plane at the point. The anisotropic Gaussian field centered at the ith point is then defined by

$$G_i(\sigma_{i_X}, X)G_i(\sigma_{i_Y}, Y)G_i(\sigma_{i_Z}, Z). \tag{5}$$

Anisotropic fields have been used in surface recovery before, but the advantage of the proposed method is the ability to adapt the overall field to the local density and organization of points. The surface normal at a point, if not given, can be estimated. For each point $\mathbf{p}_i$, the n closest points can be found and the covariance or inertia matrix $\mathbf{M}_i$ from the points can be calculated [4]. The eigenvectors of $\mathbf{M}_i$ define three orthogonal axes, which are taken as the local XYZ coordinate system at $\mathbf{p}_i$. The eigenvector associated with the smallest eigenvalue, λ_3, represents the surface normal at $\mathbf{p}_i$. The inside/outside ambiguity can be resolved by one of the existing methods [4]. Now, consider centering an anisotropic Gaussian field at $\mathbf{p}_i$ in such a way that the standard deviations of the 1-D Gaussians along the three axes are proportional to the three eigenvalues of $\mathbf{M}_i$. The Z-axis of the coordinate system of a Gaussian field represents the estimated surface normal and the X- and Y-axes represent the surface tangent at $\mathbf{p}_i$. The sum of such fields will be:

$$f_3(x, y, z) = \sum_{i=1}^{N} G_i(\sigma_{i_X}, X)G_i(\sigma_{i_Y}, Y)G_i(\sigma_{i_Z}, Z). \tag{6}$$

In order to make the parameters of the anisotropic Gaussian centered at $\mathbf{p}_i$ reflect the shape of the surface there, we estimate the principal curvatures of the surface at $\mathbf{p}_i$ and let the standard deviations of the 1-D Gaussians be inversely proportional to the curvatures. That can be accomplished by 1) fitting a bicubic polynomial to $\mathbf{p}_i$ and the n points closest to it by the weighted least-squares method with a Gaussian weight of standard deviation equal to the average distance of the n points to $\mathbf{p}_i$, 2) deriving the principal curvatures of the polynomial, and 3) evaluating them at the origin [7]. In order to smooth more in low curvature areas than in high curvature areas, the standard deviations of the 1-D Gaussians in the tangent direction are set inversely proportional to the local principal curvatures as:

$$\sigma_{i_X} = a/(1 + |\kappa_{min}|); \sigma_{i_Y} = a/(1 + |\kappa_{max}|); \sigma_{i_Z} = b\lambda_3; \tag{7}$$

that automatically adapts local smoothing to local curvature. The parameter a is a global parameter that can be varied to produce surfaces at different levels of detail. By making σ_{i_Z} proportional to λ_3, the surface smoothes more in the direction of the surface normal in areas with a higher density of points. The global smoothing in the normal direction is controlled by parameter b. Please note that parameters $\sigma_{i_X}, \sigma_{i_Y}$, and σ_{i_Z} are local to point $\mathbf{p}_i$ and vary from point to point. Therefore, the surface to be recovered consists of points where function $f_3(x, y, z)$ becomes locally maximum in the direction of surface normal. To simplify the surface recovery process, rather than finding local maxima of

$f_3(x, y, z)$, the zero-crossings of the first derivative of $f_3(x, y, z)$ in the direction of surface normal can be used:

$$f(x, y, z) = \sum_{i=1}^{N} G_i(\sigma_{i_X}, X) G_i(\sigma_{i_Y}, Y) G_i'(\sigma_{i_Z}, Z) \tag{8}$$

as the approximating surface, where $G_i'(\sigma_{i_Z}, Z)$ is the first derivative of 1-D Gaussian along the Z-axis. The zero-crossings of the resulting volume can be extracted using the marching cubes algorithm [10].

3   Results

TBI is classified into mild, moderate, or severe depending on initial assessment of responsiveness to different verbal and mental stimuli. Patients with severe TBI are usually hospitalized; their diagnosis is relatively easy as they are often unconscious. The difficulty is in identifying and differentiating patients with mild and moderate TBI, as they represent the majority of the affected population. Mild TBI patients are also those who could recover with a proper treatment, but it is very difficult to differentiate them from normal controls. Furthermore, the small amount of structural atrophy makes monitoring of mild TBI really difficult. Highly accurate ground truth data needs to be generated in order to create/evaluate fully automatic segmentation tools capable of picking up such subtle structural changes.

The described framework was used in a clinical setting to generate ground truth segmentation of the brainstem, caudate, cerebellum, corpus callosum, hippocampus, putamen, and thalamus for a set of 42 patients. The goal of our study was to identify existing structural atrophy and to generate accurate ground truth data for two different age-matched groups: healthy controls (n=18) and mild TBI (n=16). The remaining (n=8) control patients were used for reliability analysis as explained below. Obtained volumes were grouped per structure and an independent samples T-test was applied to each group. Bilateral significant differences were detected in the caudate and thalamus as illustrated in Figure 3.

An important source of error in manual expert neuro segmentation is introduced by the tracers and their ability to accurately identify and delineate the boundary of structures. In order to evaluate our approach, a subset of images (n=8) were manually traced by two different experienced tracers. The intraclass correlation coefficient (ICC) has been used as a measure of user reliability [11]. It can be interpreted as the similarity of different tracings for the same structure in terms of volume. The average absolute volume difference per structure and the average mean and root mean squared distance between closest points on corresponding spline contours placed by the two different tracers were measured as well. Results per structure are summarized in Table 1. According to the current practice, an ICC of 0.8 (80%) and above, is considered as a reliable result. Closer examination of Table 1 reveals that the presented methodology yields reliable and reproducible results with a sub-millimeter tracing error.

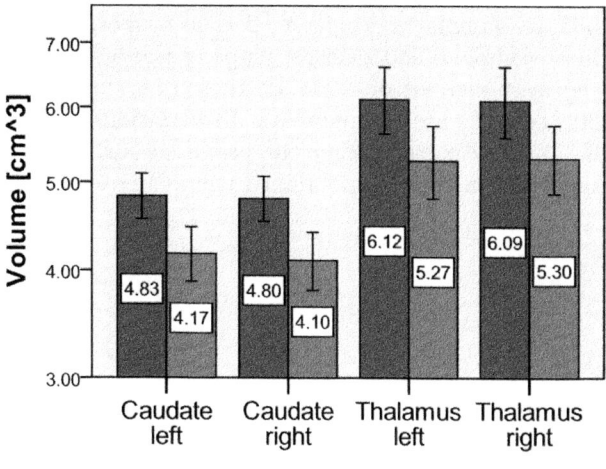

Error Bars: +/- 2 SE

Fig. 3. Statistically significant differences detected in the mild TBI patients (green) vs. controls (blue). Calculations were performed with IBM SPSS and a 95% confidence interval. p values of: .003,.002,.019,.030 were obtained for the left and right caudate and the left and right thalamus, respectively.

Table 1. The table summarizes the ICC, the average absolute volume difference, and the average mean and root mean squared distance between corresponding spline contours, per structure

	ICC		Volume [cm^3]		Mean [mm]		RMSE [mm]	
Structure	Left	Right	Left	Right	Left	Right	Left	Right
Brainstem	0.935		0.802		0.653		0.817	
Cerebellum	0.987		2.129		1.126		1.405	
Corpus callosum	0.990		0.115		0.626		0.685	
Caudate	0.813	0.896	0.267	0.157	0.548	0.539	0.690	0.676
Putamen	0.936	0.889	0.148	0.214	0.692	0.716	0.871	0.916
Hippocampus	0.950	0.808	0.214	0.290	0.614	0.661	0.765	0.783
Thalamus	0.847	0.866	0.303	0.294	1.001	0.871	1.267	1.072

Accurate ground truth data should stay as close as possible to the spline contours placed by the tracers. In order to assess the performance of the proposed surface fitting method with respect to other existing techniques, the point set illustrated in Figure 4(b) was obtained from the MR volume shown in Figure 4(a) as described above. Qualitative visual comparison of the reconstructed brainstem with the Gaussian splatter of Schroeder et al. [10], the surface reconstruction of Hoppe et al. [4], the Poisson surface reconstruction of Kazdhan et al. [5], the robust implicit moving least squares (RIMLS) method of Oztireli et al. [8], and the algebraic point set surface (APSS) of Guennebaud and Gross [3] is illustrated in Figures 4(c)-(h). The average mean and root mean squared distance between closest points on the reconstructed surface and the spline contours were evaluated as well. Results are summarized in Table 2. The proposed method was able to recover the most complete and realistic shape of the brainstem from the point cloud with the least amount of error. Furthermore, since errors from surface reconstruction (Table 2) are comparable with variations between two different tracers (Table 1), it is expected that the proposed surface reconstruction will not have a significant influence on obtained volume measurements.

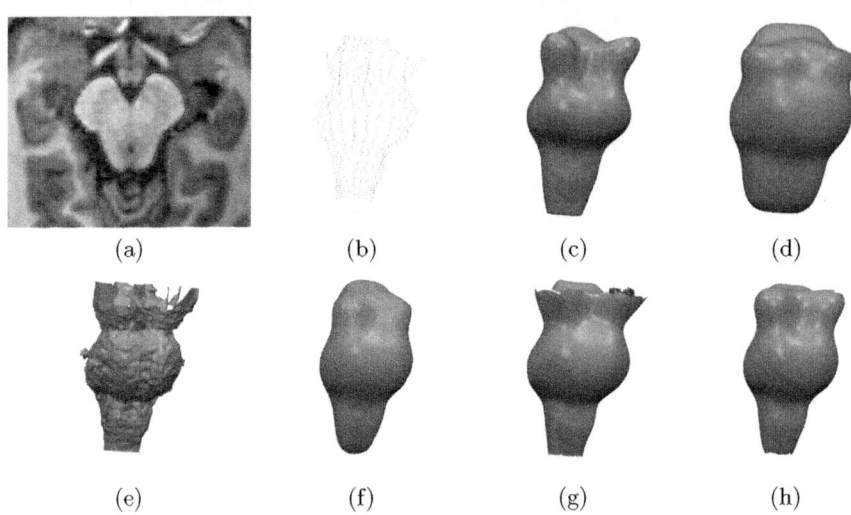

(a)   (b)   (c)   (d)

(e)   (f)   (g)   (h)

Fig. 4. (a) An axial slice from an MR volume with initialized control points on the boundary of the brainstem. (b) The point set obtained by combining sampled spline points from all slices. The brainstem surface obtained by (c) the proposed, (d) splatter, (e) surface reconstruction, (f) Poisson, (g) RIMLS, and (h) APSS methods. The proposed method has been able to recover the most complete shape of the brainstem.

Table 2. The mean and root mean squared distance between recovered surface and spline points for the different surface reconstruction methods

	Proposed	Splatter	SRecon	Poisson	RIMLS	APSS
Mean	0.679	6.019	1.725	1.436	1.692	1.461
RMSE	0.847	6.120	2.423	1.611	1.947	1.718

4   Conclusion

Tracers were allowed to initialize and edit planar B-spline curves, delineating the boundary of brain structures on consecutive MR slices. Volumetric representations of traced structures were extracted from the B-spline curves in the form of 3-D point clouds. A new implicit surface formulation was developed and used to recover an explicit boundary surface of the corresponding 3-D point clouds.

Experimental results demonstrate that complex geometries can be recovered. The tracing is accurate, the approach was able to identify subtle atrophy of brain structures known to be implicated in mild TBI, which is still a challenge. Intraclass correlation of results from different tracers also indicates that reliable segmentation can be accomplished. That, coupled with the ease of editing, makes the proposed approach much more attractive for accurate ground truth annotation as opposed to manual bitmask drawing. Most importantly, it provides a viable methodology for the generation of accurate ground truth data needed for the training of many fully-automatic techniques.

References

1. Barnes, J., Foster, J., Boyes, R., Pepple, T., Moore, E., Schott, J., Frost, C., Scahill, R., Fox, N.: A comparison of methods for the automated calculation of volumes and atrophy rates in the hippocampus. Neuroimage 40(4), 1655–1671 (2008)
2. Fischl, B., Salat, D., Busa, E., Albert, M., Dieterich, M., Haselgrove, C., van der Kouwe, A., Killiany, R., Kennedy, D., Klaveness, S., et al.: Whole brain segmentation automated labeling of neuroanatomical structures in the human brain. Neuron 33(3), 341–355 (2002)
3. Guennebaud, G., Gross, M.: Algebraic point set surfaces. In: ACM SIGGRAPH, pp. 23–31. ACM Press, New York (2007)
4. Hoppe, H., DeRose, T., Duchamp, T., McDonald, J., Stuetzle, W.: Surface reconstruction from unorganized points. In: Proc. SIGGRAPH, pp. 163–169 (1992)
5. Kazhdan, M., Bolitho, M., Hoppe, H.: Poisson surface reconstruction. In: Polthier, K., Sheffer, A. (eds.) Eurographics Symposium on Geometry Processing. ACM Press, New York (2006)
6. Morey, R., Petty, C., Xu, Y., Pannu Hayes, J., Wagner, H., Lewis, D., LaBar, K., Styner, M., McCarthy, G.: A comparison of automated segmentation and manual tracing for quantifying hippocampal and amygdala volumes. NeuroImage 45(3), 855–866 (2009)
7. Mortenson, M.E.: Geometric Modeling. Wiley Press, New York (1985)
8. Oztireli, A., Guennebaud, G., Gross, M.: Feature preserving point set surfaces based on non-linear kernel regression. Computer Graphics Forum 28(2), 493–501 (2009)
9. Patenaude, B., Smith, S., Kennedy, D., Jenkinson, M.: First-fmrib's integrated registration and segmentation tool. In: Human Brain Mapping Conference (2007)
10. Schroeder, W., Martin, K., Lorensen, B.: The Visualization Toolkit, 3rd edn. Kitware Inc. (2004)
11. Shrout, P., Fleiss, J.: Intraclass correlations: uses in assessing rater reliability. Psychol. Bull. 86(2), 420–428 (1979)

Multi-Modal Multi-Task Learning for Joint Prediction of Clinical Scores in Alzheimer's Disease

Daoqiang Zhang[1,2] and Dinggang Shen[1]

[1] Dept. of Radiology and BRIC, University of North Carolina at Chapel Hill, NC 27599
[2] Dept. of Computer Science and Engineering, Nanjing University of Aeronautics and
Astronautics, Nanjing 210016, China
{zhangd,dgshen}@med.unc.edu

Abstract. One recent interest in computer-aided diagnosis of neurological
diseases is to predict the clinical scores from brain images. Most existing
methods usually estimate multiple clinical variables separately, without
considering the useful correlation information among them. On the other hand,
nearly all methods use only one modality of data (mostly structural MRI) for
regression, and thus ignore the complementary information among different
modalities. To address these issues, in this paper, we present a general
methodology, namely Multi-Modal Multi-Task (M3T) learning, to jointly
predict multiple variables from multi-modal data. Our method contains three
major subsequent steps: (1) a multi-task feature selection which selects the
common subset of relevant features for the related multiple clinical variables
from each modality; (2) a kernel-based multimodal data fusion which fuses the
above-selected features from all modalities; (3) a support vector regression
which predicts multiple clinical variables based on the previously learnt mixed
kernel. Experimental results on ADNI dataset with both imaging modalities
(MRI and PET) and biological modality (CSF) validate the efficacy of the
proposed M3T learning method.

1 Introduction

Alzheimer's disease (AD) is the most common form of dementia in elderly people
worldwide. Over the past decades, many AD classification methods have been
developed for early diagnosis of AD (including its prodromal stage, i.e., mild
cognitive impairment (MCI)) [1-5]. Recently, some AD regression methods are also
proposed for the prediction of clinical scores based on brain images [6-9]. Compared
with classification, regression needs to estimate continuous rather than categorical
variables and are thus more challenging. On the other hand, accurate estimation of
clinical scores from brain images is important for helping evaluate the stage of AD
pathology and predicting future progression.

In practical diagnosis of AD, generally multiple clinical scores are acquired, i.e.,
Mini Mental State Examination (MMSE) and Alzheimer's Disease Assessment Scale-
Cognitive subtest (ADAS-Cog). Specifically, MMSE examines the orientation to time
and place, the immediate and delayed recall of three words, the attention and
calculations, language, and visuoconstructional functions, while ADAS-Cog is a

T. Liu et al. (Eds.): MBIA 2011, LNCS 7012, pp. 60–67, 2011.

global measure encompassing the core symptoms of AD [8]. It is known that there exist inherent correlations among multiple clinical scores of a subject, since the underlying pathology is the same. However, most existing methods model different clinical scores separately, without considering their inherent correlations that may be useful for robust and accurate estimation of clinical scores from brain images. Recently, a few studies on joint estimation of multiple clinical variables have appeared in imaging literature. For example, in [9], the authors assumed that the related clinical scores share a common relevant feature subset. However, for obtaining a common relevant feature subset, they still needed to perform separate feature selection for each clinical score, and then concatenated the same number of top-ranked features from each clinical score to build a joint regression model.

On the other hand, although multi-modal data are usually acquired for AD diagnosis, i.e., MRI, PET, and CSF biomarkers, nearly all the regression methods developed for estimation of clinical scores were based only on one imaging modality, i.e., the structural MRI. Recent studies have indicated that the biomarkers from different modalities provide complementary information, which is very useful for AD diagnosis [3]. More recently, a series of research works have started to use multi-modal data for AD classification and obtained the improved performance compared with the methods based only on single-modal data [4-5]. However, to the best of our knowledge, the same type of study in imaging-based regression, i.e., estimation of clinical scores from multi-modal data, was not investigated previously.

Inspired by the above problems, in this paper, we present a general methodology, namely Multi-Modal Multi-Task (M3T) learning, to jointly predict multiple clinical scores from multi-modal data. Here, we treat the estimations of multiple clinical scores as different tasks. Specifically, at first, as in the conventional multi-task feature learning methods [10-12], we assume that the related tasks share a common relevant feature subset but with a varying amount of influence on each task, and adopt a multi-task feature selection method [10-11] to obtain a common feature subset for different tasks simultaneously. Then, we use a kernel-based multimodal-data-fusion method to fuse the above-selected features from each individual modality. Finally, we use a support vector regression method [13] to predict multiple clinical scores based on the previously-learnt mixed kernel.

The rest of this paper is organized as follows. In Section 2, we present the proposed Multi-Modal Multi-Task (M3T) learning method in detail. Section 3 reports the experimental results on ADNI dataset using MRI, PET, and CSF biomarkers. Finally, we conclude this paper and indicate issues for future work in Section 4.

2   Method

In this section, we present the new Multi-Modal Multi-Task (M3T) learning method. Our method consists of three subsequent steps, i.e., multi-task feature selection, multiple-modal data fusion, and support vector regression. Specifically, we first assume that the related tasks share a common relevant feature subset but with varying amount of influence on each task, and adopt a multi-task feature selection method to obtain a common feature subset for different tasks simultaneously. Then, we use the kernel-based multimodal-data-fusion method to fuse the above-selected features from each individual modality. Finally, we use a support vector regression to predict multiple clinical scores based on the previously-learnt mixed kernel. Fig. 1 illustrates the flowchart of the proposed M3T method. Note that the feature extraction from MRI and PET images will be discussed in the next section.

2.1   Multi-Task Feature Selection

For imaging modalities such as MRI and PET, even after feature extraction, the number of features (extracted from brain regions) may be still large. Besides, not all features are relevant to the diseases, i.e., clinical scores (tasks). So, feature selection is commonly used for dimensionality reduction, as well as for removal of irrelevant features. Different from the conventional single-task feature selection, the multi-task feature selection simultaneously selects a common feature subset relevant to all tasks [10]. This point is especially important for diagnosis of neurological diseases, since multiple clinical scores are essentially determined by the same underlying pathology, i.e., the diseased brain regions. On the other hand, simultaneously performing feature selection for multiple clinical variables is also very helpful to suppress the noises in the individual clinical scores.

Suppose that we have N training subjects with M modalities and T tasks (clinical scores). Let $x_i^{(1)},..., x_i^{(M)}$ denote the M modalities of data and $t_i^{(1)},..., t_i^{(T)}$ the responses of T different tasks for the i-th subject, respectively. Denote $A^{(m)} = [x_1^{(m)}, ..., x_N^{(m)}]^T$ as the training data matrix on the m-th modality and $y^{(j)} = [t_1^{(j)}, ..., t_N^{(j)}]^T$ as the response vector on the j-th task, respectively. Following [10-11], linear models are used to model the multi-task feature selection (MTFS) as:

$$\hat{t}^{(j)}(x^{(m)}, w_j^{(m)}) = \left(x^{(m)}\right)^T w_j^{(m)}, \quad j = 1,...,T, m = 1,...,M , \tag{1}$$

where $w_j^{(m)}$ is the weight vector for the j-th task on m-th modality. The weight vectors for all T tasks form a weight matrix $W^{(m)} = [w_1^{(m)}, ..., w_T^{(m)}]$, which can be optimized by the following objective function:

$$\begin{aligned}\min_{W^{(m)}} \quad &\frac{1}{2}\sum_{j=1}^{T}\sum_{i=1}^{N}\left(t_i^{(j)} - \hat{t}^{(j)}(x_i^{(m)}, w_j^{(m)})\right)^2 + \lambda \sum_{d=1}^{D_m}\left\|(w^d)^{(m)}\right\|_2 \\ = &\frac{1}{2}\sum_{j=1}^{T}\left\|y^{(j)} - A^{(m)} w_j^{(m)}\right\|_2^2 + \lambda \sum_{d=1}^{D_m}\left\|(w^d)^{(m)}\right\|_2\end{aligned} \tag{2}$$

where $(w^d)^{(m)}$ denotes the d-th row of $W^{(m)}$, D_m is the dimension of the m-th modal data, and λ is the regularization coefficient controlling the relative contributions of the two terms. Note that λ also controls the 'sparsity' of the linear models, with the high value corresponding to more sparse models (i.e., more values in $W^{(m)}$ are zero). It is easy to know that Eq. 2 reduces to the standard l_1-norm regularized optimization problem in Lasso [14] when there is only one task. In our case, this is actually a multi-task learning for given m-th modal data.

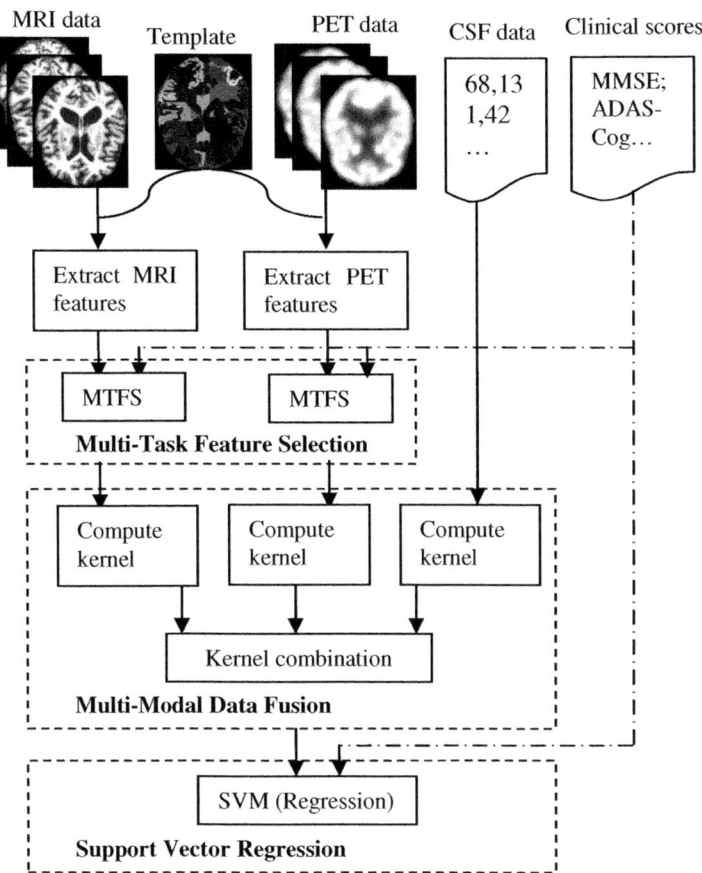

Fig. 1. Flowchart of the proposed M3T method

The key point of Eq. 2 is the use of l_2-norm for $(w^d)^{(m)}$, which forces the weights corresponding to the d-th feature (of the m-th modal data) across multiple tasks to be grouped together and tends to select features based on the strength of T tasks jointly. Note that, because of the characteristic of 'group sparsity', the solution of Eq. 2 results in a weight matrix $W^{(m)}$ whose elements in some rows are all zeros [11]. For feature selection, we just keep those features with non-zero weights. At present, there are many algorithms developed to solve Eq. 2, and in this paper we adopt the SLEP toolbox [15], which has been shown very effective on many datasets.

2.2 Multi-Modal Data Fusion

To effectively fuse data from different modalities, we adopt a multiple-kernels combination scheme in this paper. Assume that we have N training subjects, and each subject has M modalities of data, represented as $x_i=\{x_i^{(1)},\dots, x_i^{(m)},\dots, x_i^{(M)}\}$, $i=1,\dots,N$ (similar to those defined above). Let $k^{(m)}(.,.)$ denote the kernel function on the m-th modality, and then we can define the kernel function $k(.,.)$ on two data x and z as:

$$k(x, z) = \sum_{m=1}^{M} \beta_m k^{(m)}(x^{(m)}, z^{(m)}), \tag{3}$$

Where β_ms are the nonnegative weight parameters used to balance the contributions of different modalities. All β_ms are constrained by $\sum_m \beta_m = 1$.

Once we have defined the kernel function $k(., .)$ on multimodal data, a N by N kernel matrix K on multimodal data of all training subjects can be straightforwardly obtained as $K = \{k(x_i, x_j)\}$. Then, the subsequent learner such as support vector regression (SVR) can be directly built with the kernel matrix K.

2.3   Support Vector Regression

After obtaining a common feature subset for all different tasks by MTFS and then using those selected features to generate the mixed kernel matrix through multimodal data fusion, we can now train the support vector regression (SVR) to get the final regression models. Here, for simplicity of implementation, we train a separate SVR model for each task. However, it is worth noting that, since we use the common subset of features (selected by MTFS during the feature selection stage) to train the regression models, our models are actually multi-task learning methods, rather than single-task ones. Moreover, one advantage of our models is that they can be easily solved by the standard SVM solvers, e.g., LIBSVM [16].

3   Experiments

In this section, we evaluate the effectiveness of the proposed method for Multi-Modal Multi-Task learning on the Alzheimer's Disease Neuroimaging Initiative (ADNI) database (www.loni.ucla.edu/ADNI). In our experiments, we use three modalities of data including MRI, PET and CSF data. On the other hand, we use two clinical scores, i.e., MMSE and ADAS-Cog, as the two related tasks.

3.1   Subjects and Settings

The ADNI database contains approximately 200 cognitively normal elderly subjects to be followed for 3 years, 400 subjects with MCI to be followed for 3 years, and 200 subjects with early AD to be followed for 2 years. In this paper, all ADNI baseline subjects with the corresponding MRI, PET, and CSF data are included. This yields a total of 202 subjects, including 51 AD patients, 99 MCI patients, and 52 healthy controls. Standard image pre-processing is performed for all MRI and PET images, including anterior commissure (AC) - posterior commissure (PC) correction, skull-stripping, removal of cerebellum, and segmentation of structural MR images into three different tissues: grey matter (GM), white matter (WM), and cerebrospinal fluid (CSF). With atlas warping, we can partition each subject image into 93 regions of interests (ROIs). For each of the 93 ROIs, we compute the GM tissue volume from the subject's MRI image. For PET image, we first rigidly align it with its respective MRI image of the same subject, and then compute the average value of PET signals in each ROI. Therefore, for each subject, we can finally obtain totally 93 features from MRI image, other 93 features from PET image, and 3 features ($A\beta_{42}$, t-tau, and p-tau) from CSF biomarkers.

In our experiments, we compare our Multi-Modal Multi-Task learning method (denoted as M3T) with conventional Single-Modal Single-Task learning method (denoted as SMST). In SMST, a single-task feature selection (Eq. 2 with single task, i.e., Lasso) is first adopted to select the relevant features for each task separately, and then SVR is performed on those selected features. For comparison, we also implement two other variants, i.e., Single-Modal Multi-Task (SMMT) and Multi-Modal Single-Task (MMST) learning methods. Compared with M3T, single task feature selection (Lasso) is used in MMST, and a single-kernel SVR is used in SMMT. It is worth noting that neither method has been used for regression of clinical scores previously. In addition, we also compare M3T with a Recursive Feature Elimination (RFE) based feature selection also used for joint regression of multiple clinical scores [9], where for fair comparison, we implement the same procedure for the feature selection as in [9] and then use SVR for regression as in our method; we denote this method as RFE_SVR.

Five-fold cross-validation is adopted to evaluate the performances of different algorithms for estimation of multiple clinical scores by measuring the correlation coefficient between the actual clinical score and the predicted one [8]. For all respective methods, the values of the parameters (e.g., λ and β) are determined by performing another cross-validation on the training data. Also, linear kernel is used in SVR after performing a common feature normalization step, i.e., subtracting the mean and then dividing the standard deviation across all subjects for each feature value.

3.2   Results

Table 1 shows the comparison results on regression performances of five different methods. Here, for the multi-task methods (SMMT and M3T), we use the original features of CSF rather than the selected features by feature selection step, since there are only 3 features in this modality.

As can be seen from Table 1, the proposed M3T method is always superior to the conventional SMST method. Specifically, for the estimation of MMSE score, M3T achieves the highest correlation (0.532), while the best corresponding result of SMST is only 0.479 (on MRI modality); on the other hand, for the estimation of ADAS-Cog score, M3T achieves the highest correlation (0.598), while the best corresponding result of SMST is 0.577 (on PET modality). A closer observation on Table 1 shows that the performances of MMST are consistently better than those of other methods except M3T. This validates our assumption that the complementary information among different modalities is helpful for regression, which complements a similar well-known conclusion for classification. Furthermore, by simultaneously using multi-modal and multi-task information, M3T always achieves the best performance among all methods. On the other hand, Table 1 shows RFE_SVR is inferior to M3T which validates the advantage of multi-task feature selection over the strategy of concatenating features from separate single-task feature selection.

Finally, Fig. 2 shows the scatter plots of predicted clinical scores vs. actual scores by two methods for MMSE and ADAS-Cog, respectively. Here, due to space limit, we only list the results of SMST (on MRI modality) and M3T. As can be seen from Fig. 2, using multi-modal and multi-task information in M3T achieves better results than conventional SMST method.

Table 1. Comparison on regression performances of different methods. The reported values are correlation coefficients (mean ± standard deviation).

Methods	Modality	Task 1 (MMSE)	Task 2 (ADAS-cog)
SMST	MRI	0.479±0.112	0.433±0.164
	CSF	0.351±0.105	0.346±0.109
	PET	0.389±0.101	0.577±0.143
MMST	Multi-modal	0.513±0.078	0.581±0.148
SMMT	MRI	0.483±0.122	0.469±0.160
	CSF	0.351±0.105	0.346±0.109
	PET	0.409±0.116	0.580±0.147
M3T	Multi-modal	0.532±0.097	0.598±0.145
RFE_SVR	MRI	0.507±0.114	0.483±0.180

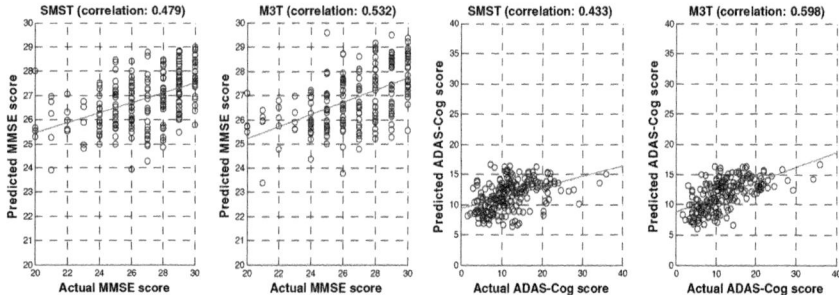

Fig. 2. Scatter plots of predicted **MMSE** and **ADAS-Cog** scores vs. actual scores by SMST (column 1 and 3) and M3T (column 2 and 4). The red solid lines represent the regression lines.

4   Conclusion

We have formulized a new learning problem, called Multi-Modal Multi-Task (M3T) learning, which originates naturally from the practical neurological diseases. Then, we use a new learning framework to jointly predict multiple clinical scores for AD. Specifically, we have developed a new method by combining multi-task feature selection, kernel-based multi-modal data fusion, and support vector regression within an integrated framework. Experimental results on the ADNI dataset have validated the efficacy of the Multi-Modal Multi-Task learning method. In future work, we will develop models which can iteratively use the multi-modal and multi-task information rather than the sequential combination in this paper to further improve performances.

Acknowledgments. This work was supported in part by NIH grants EB006733, EB008374, EB009634 and MH088520, and also by National Science Foundation of China under grant No. 60875030.

References

1. Kloppel, S., Stonnington, C.M., Chu, C., Draganski, B., Scahill, R.I., Rohrer, J.D., Fox, N.C., Jack Jr., C.R., Ashburner, J., Frackowiak, R.S.: Automatic classification of MR scans in Alzheimer's disease. Brain 131, 681–689 (2008)
2. Vemuri, P., Wiste, H.J., Weigand, S.D., Shaw, L.M., Trojanowski, J.Q., Weiner, M.W., Knopman, D.S., Petersen, R.C., Jack Jr., C.R.: MRI and CSF biomarkers in normal, MCI, and AD subjects: predicting future clinical change. Neurology 73, 294–301 (2009)
3. Walhovd, K.B., Fjell, A.M., Dale, A.M., McEvoy, L.K., Brewer, J., Karow, D.S., Salmon, D.P., Fennema-Notestine, C.: Multi-modal imaging predicts memory performance in normal aging and cognitive decline. Neurobiol. Aging 31, 1107–1121 (2010)
4. Hinrichs, C., Singh, V., Xu, G., Johnson, S.: MKL for robust multi-modality AD classification. Med. Image Comput. Comput. Assist. Interv. 12, 786–794 (2009)
5. Ye, J., Chen, K., Wu, T., Li, J., Zhao, Z., Patel, R., Bae, M., Janardan, R., Liu, H., Alexander, G., Reiman, E.M.: Heterogeneous data fusion for Alzheimer's disease study. In: ACM International Conference on Knowledge Discovery and Data Mining (2008)
6. Duchesne, S., Caroli, A., Geroldi, C., Frisoni, G.B., Collins, D.L.: Predicting clinical variable from MRI features: Application to MMSE in MCI. In: Duncan, J.S., Gerig, G. (eds.) MICCAI 2005. LNCS, vol. 3749, pp. 392–399. Springer, Heidelberg (2005)
7. Wang, Y., Fan, Y., Bhatt, P., Davatzikos, C.: High-dimensional pattern regression using machine learning: from medical images to continuous variables. NeuroImage 50, 1519–1535 (2010)
8. Stonnington, C.M., Chu, C., Kloppel, S., Jack Jr., C.R., Ashburner, J., Frackowiak, R.S.J.: Predicting clinical scores from magnetic resonance scans in Alzheimer's disease. NeuroImage 51, 1405–1413 (2010)
9. Fan, Y., Kaufer, D., Shen, D.: Joint estimation of multiple clinical variables of neurological diseases from imaging patterns. In: The 2010 IEEE International Conference on Biomedical Imaging: from Nano to Macro, pp. 852–855 (2010)
10. Obozinski, G., Taskar, B., Jordan, M.I.: Multi-task feature selection. Technical report, Statistics Department, UC Berkeley (2006)
11. Liu, J., Ji, S., Ye, J.: Multi-task feature learning via efficient l2,1-norm minimization. In: Uncertainty in Artificial Intelligence (2009)
12. Yang, X., Kim, S., Xing, E.P.: Heterogeneous multitask learning with joint sparsity constraints. In: Advances in Neural Information Processing Systems (2009)
13. Vapnik, V.: Statistical Learning Theory. Wiley, New York (1998)
14. Tibshirani, R.: Regression shrinkage and selection via the lasso. Journal of the Royal Statistical Society Series B 58, 267–288 (1996)
15. Liu, J., Ji, S., Ye, J.: SLEP: Sparse Learning with Efficient Projections. Technical report, Arizona State University (2009)
16. Chang, C.C., Lin, C.J.: LIBSVM: a library for support vector machines (2001)

Identification of Cortical Landmarks Based on Consistent Connectivity to Subcortical Structures

Degang Zhang[1,3], Lei Guo[1], Dajiang Zhu[2], Tuo Zhang[1], Xintao Hu[1], Kaiming Li[1,2],
Xi Jiang[2], Hanbo Chen[2], Jinglei Lv[1], Fan Deng[2], and Qun Zhao[3]

[1] School of Automation, Northwestern Polytechnical University, Xi'an, China
[2] Department of Computer Science and Bioimaging Research Center,
The University of Georgia, Athens, GA
[3] Department of Physics and Bioimaging Research Center, The University
of Georgia, Athens, GA, United States

Abstract. Quantitative assessment of structural connectivities between cortical and subcortical regions has been of increasing interest in recent years. This paper proposes an algorithmic pipeline for identification of reliable cortical landmarks based on the consistent structural connectivity between cortical and subcortical regions. First, twelve subcortical regions are segmented from MRI data, and cortical surface and white matter fibers are reconstructed and tracked from magnetic resonance diffusion tensor imaging (DTI) data. Second, given that subcortical structures are relatively consistent across individual subjects, the structural connectivity from cortical to subcortical regions is extracted as the connectional attribute for each cortical region. Third, the cortex is segmented into different regions based on their cortico-subcortical connection attributes, and regions with the most consistent connectivity patterns across different subjects are selected as cortical landmarks. Experimental results from eight healthy subjects show that our approaches can identify 22 reliable cortical landmarks, a portion of which are validated via task-based fMRI data.

Keywords: cortical parcellation, subcortical regions, connectivity pattern.

1 Introduction

It has been widely recognized that each brain's cytoarchitectonic area has a unique set of extrinsic inputs and outputs, and this is crucial in determining the functions that the area can perform [1]. This unique set of brain connectivity patterns is called 'connectional fingerprint' [1]. The hypothesis of unique connectional fingerprints was supported by statistical analyses of cortical connectivity in primate [2] and feline cortex [3]. In the brain imaging community, the concept of connectional fingerprint has been utilized for *in vivo* parcellation of the cerebral cortex. For instance, it was reported in [4] that connectivity patterns of cortical regions to the thalamus nuclei can be used to parcellate the cortex into different meaningful sub-regions.

In this paper, we utilize the structural connectivity between cortical and subcortical regions to segment cortical areas based on the following two rationales. 1) Subcortical regions including amygdala, hippocampus, thalamus, caudate, putamen, and globus pallidus, have been shown to be relatively reliable and consistent across individual brains [5], and current segmentation approaches can achieve satisfactory segmentation results [6]. Given the remarkable variability of cortical anatomy, these reliable and

T. Liu et al. (Eds.): MBIA 2011, LNCS 7012, pp. 68–75, 2011.

consistent subcortical regions can serve as the reliable reference landmarks for the definition of structural connectivity features. 2) Instead of using a single subcortical region, e.g., in [4], we use 6 subcortical regions (in each hemisphere) as a reference system to define the cortico-subcortical structural connectivity pattern for a cortical area. This systematic exploration of the connectivity pattern between cortical and subcortical regions provides us a rich information source for identifying meaningful boundaries between cortical regions.

2 Methods

2.1 Overview, Data Acquisition and Preprocessing

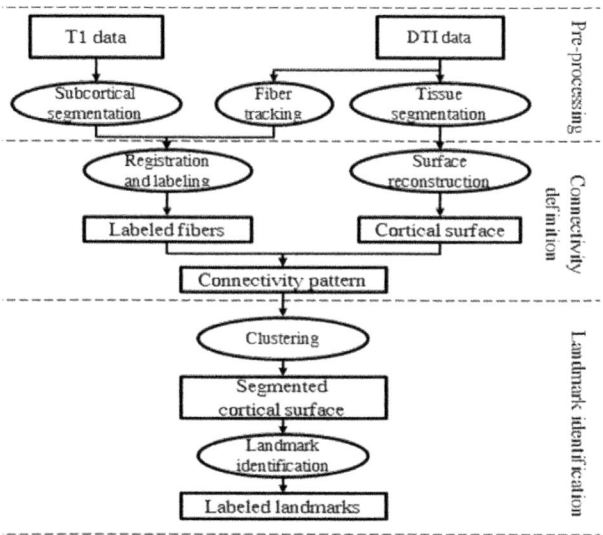

Fig. 1. The flowchart of the proposed framework

The flowchart of the proposed cortical landmark identification approach based on cortico-subcortical connectivity patterns is illustrated in Fig. 1. The algorithmic pipeline is composed of three major phases. The preprocessing phase includes: segmentation of subcortical regions from T1 data, brain tissue segmentation from DTI data, and DTI tractography. The second phase of defining cortico-subcortical connectivity attribute includes: reconstruction of cortical surface from DTI data, labeling the cortico-subcortical connection fibers into clusters based on the anatomical locations of their end points, and definition and examination of cortico-subcortical connection patterns. The third phase of landmark identification identifies consistent cortical regions based on the consistency of cortico-subcortical connection patterns across different subjects.

Eight healthy volunteers were scanned in a 3T GE MRI system with institutional review board (IRB) approval. 3D T1 SPGR images were collected for subcortical segmentation and spatial co-registration. DTI data were acquired with dimensionality of 128×128×60 and isotropic special resolution of 2mm×2mm×2mm. Parameters were TR 15.5s and TE 89.5ms, with 30 diffusion weighted gradient directions and 3 B0 volumes acquired. Pre-processing steps included brain skull removal, motion correction, and eddy current correction [8]. After the pre-processing, we performed fiber tracking, white matter (WM) segmentation, and cortical surface reconstruction based on the DTI data [9]. Fiber tracking was performed using MEDINRIA. Based on the WM segmentation, the cortical surface was reconstructed using similar methods in [7]. The surface has about 40,000 vertices. The FSL tools [6] were used for preprocessing and subcortical regions segmentation of the T1 images. The subcortical regions are registered to the DTI space using an affine transformation with 6 degrees of freedom (DOF).

2.2 Subcortical Region Segmentation and Fiber Labeling

We employed the FSL FIRST [10] tool to segment 12 subcortical regions from T1 MRI data. Fig. 2 shows eight examples of subcortical segmentation results. It shows that the segmented subcortical regions are quite consistent across these eight subjects. These segmented subcortical regions are warped to the DTI image space via the FSL FLIRT tool. Then, based on the white matter fibers tracked from DTI data, all of the fibers connecting subcortical and cortical regions are extracted. In particular, these extracted fibers are clustered into 12 bundles, each of which corresponds to the set of fibers connecting the same hemisphere subcortical region. For instance, Fig. 3 shows the 6 clustered bundles corresponding to the 6 subcortical regions on the right hemisphere. The colors of the bundles in Fig. 3 are in correspondences with the colors of the subcortical regions in Fig. 2.

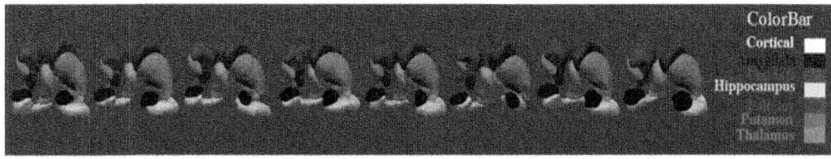

Fig. 2. The segmentation results of 12 subcortical regions in 8 subjects. The color bar is on the right side.

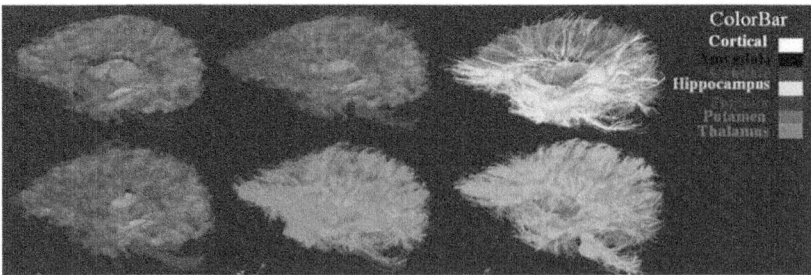

Fig. 3. Joint visualization of cortical surface, subcortical regions and the fibers for 6 subcortical regions in the right hemisphere. The color bar is shown on the right side.

2.3   Cortico-Subcortical Connectivity Patterns

In general, the segmented subcortical regions in Fig. 2 and the labeled cortico-subcortical fibers in Fig. 3 provide a set of reliable reference landmarks to define structural connectivity from the cortex to subcortical structures. That is, for any cortical region, the composition of fiber types naturally provides an intrinsic connectional fingerprint [1] to define this cortical region's structural connectivity pattern and thus reflects the function that this region performs. It should be noted that based on the segmented 12 subcortical regions from T1 MRI image in Fig. 2, we consider the connectivity between a cortical region and 6 subcortical regions on the left and right hemispheres separately, in order to facilitate algorithm development and validation at current stage. The major reason is that there is more variability and inaccuracy for the DTI streamline tractography algorithm to track cross-hemisphere cortico-subcortical fibers, which will increase the inconsistency of connection patterns. Therefore, we used 6 intra-hemisphere cortico-subcortical fibers bundles for connectivity pattern definition in this paper, and we have 2^6 (64) connectivity patterns for each hemisphere respectively. Specifically, for each cortical region with a fixed size (we call it as surface patch), we search its connecting fibers' subcortical (in the same hemisphere) labels, and used these labels as the cortico-subcortical connectivity pattern. For instance, if there is any fiber that connects to a specified subcortical region, we set its item in the connectivity pattern as 1, otherwise as 0. Fig. 4 shows three examples of cortico-subcortical connection patterns.

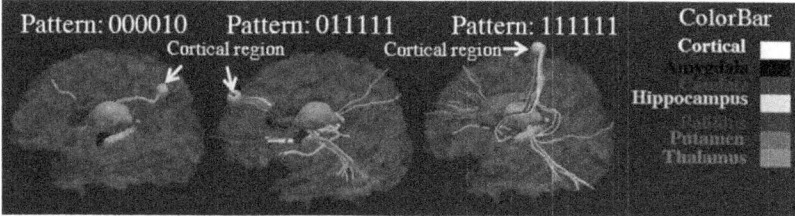

Fig. 4. Three examples of the cortico-subcortical connectivity patterns

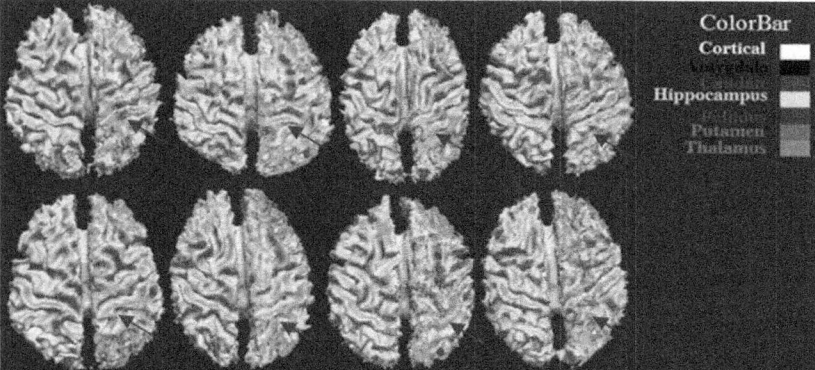

Fig. 5. Demonstration of consistent fiber composition patterns on the right hemisphere. Eight subjects are shown here. The fibers with different colors indicate different subcortical regions they connect to. The color bar is on the right.

2.4 Consistent Cortical Landmark Identification

The cerebral cortex of human brain has remarkably variable shapes across individuals. This tremendous variability renders significant challenges to human brain mapping. It is also widely recognized in the field that there is common brain architecture [1]. Our premise here is that the cortico-subcortical connection patterns are among the most reliable and consistent brain architecture. Our extensive visual observations and quantitative evaluations in this paper support the above premise, as shown in Fig. 5 as an example. The subcortical fiber composition patterns of eight subjects are shown in Fig. 5. We can see that the distributions of the subcortical fiber composition patterns in these subjects are relatively similar, e.g., the cortical regions highlighted by red arrows, suggesting the existence of common cortico-subcortical connection patterns in cortical regions. Therefore, we will extract segmented cortical regions that have consistent cortico-subcortical connection patterns across different subjects as the structural landmarks.

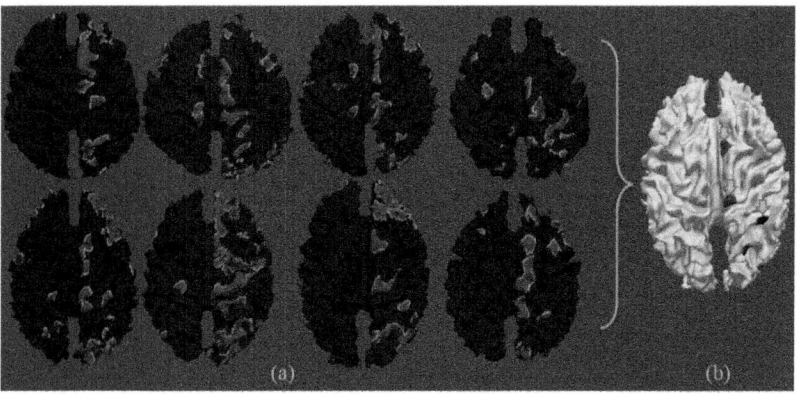

Fig. 6. Demonstration of consistent cortical landmark ROI identification based on one connectivity pattern (the cortical region is connected to all of six subcortical regions in the same hemisphere). (a): Illustration of the clustering result of one connectivity pattern of eight subjects. (b): Illustration of the consistent cortical landmark ROIs across eight subjects (highlighted by the yellow arrow as examples). The different colors of surface patches indicate different landmark ROIs on the surface.

The cortico-subcortical connectivity pattern defined in the above section is used to segment cortical regions by using vertex clustering. We simply adopted the connected component detection method to cluster cortical vertices into regions. That is, if two neighboring surface patches have the same cortico-subcortical connectivity pattern, they are linked and merged into a larger region. Each connected cortical region is separated into a single region. The clustering results of the connectivity patterns of eight subjects for one connection pattern are shown in Fig. 6(a). Once the cortical regions in individual brains are segmented, the consistency and variability of their cortico-subcortical fiber connection patterns can be quantitatively evaluated and visually inspected. That is, all fibers connecting to each labeled cortical region will be extracted for different subjects, and their connectivity pattern similarities will be quantified. The cortical regions with consistent connection patterns will be selected as cortical landmark ROIs, as shown in Fig 6(b).

3   Experimental Results

3.1   Cortical Landmark Identification

We applied the approaches in Sections 2.2-2.4 on our DTI dataset, achieving 22 reliable and consistent cortical landmarks as shown in Fig. 7. It shows that the identified cortical landmarks are quite consistently distributed over the eight cortical surfaces, suggesting the robustness and effectiveness of our methods. For instance, the landmarks highlighted by red, white and yellow arrows are consistently localized on similar cortical regions in different brains. Here the corresponding cortical landmarks in different subjects are labeled by the same colors.

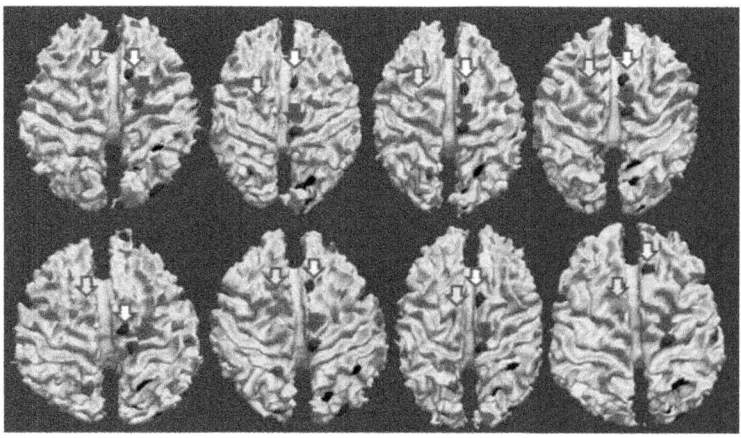

Fig. 7. 22 cortical landmarks identified by the cortico-subcortical connectivity patterns. The surface patches with same colors indicate corresponding regions across different subjects. The red, yellow and white arrows highlight corresponding cortical landmarks as examples.

3.2   Evaluation of Cortical Landmarks by Fiber Connection Patterns

In this subsection, we visually and quantitatively evaluate the cortical landmarks identified in section 3.1 by examining the consistency of the white matter fibers connected to them. For visualization purpose, we randomly selected one landmark (Figs. 8a), and extracted all of the fibers that are connected to it (Figs. 8b). In particular, we differentiated the fibers connected to this landmark into cortico-subcortical (cyan) and cortico-cortical (white) ones. It is evident that both of the cortico-subcortical and cortico-cortical fiber bundles are reasonably consistent across eight subjects. It should be noted that it is not surprising that the cortico-subcortical fiber bundles are consistent in that the cortical landmarks were identified by these consistent connection patterns. However, it is striking that the cortico-cortical fiber bundles are also quite consistent, thus offering an *independent cross-validation* to our cortical landmark identification approach. These results in Fig. 8 demonstrated the effectiveness and validity of our proposed approach for cortical landmark identification based on consistent cortico-subcortical structural connectivity patterns. Quantitatively, the average Hausdorff distances between any pairs of ROIs' fiber

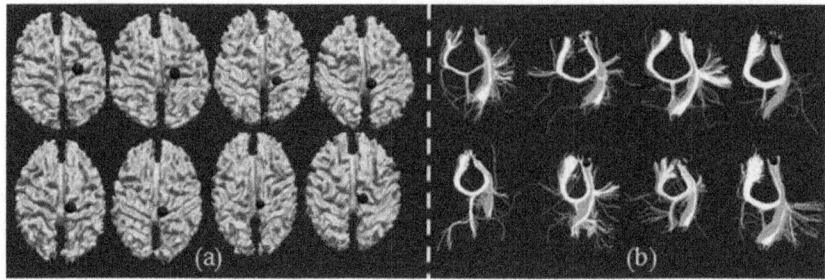

Fig. 8. Consistency evaluation of fibers connected to the second landmark in eight subjects. (a): The landmark locations are indicated by red bubbles. (b): Fibers connected to the landmarks. The cyan fibers are connections between the cortical landmark and subcortical regions, while the white fibers are connections between the cortical landmark and other cortical regions.

bundles across different subjects are 3.9 mm and 3.67 mm for the first and second landmarks respectively, which are regarded as relatively small considering results reported in the literature [11].

3.3   Validation of Cortical Landmarks via Task-Based fMRI

In order to evaluate and validate the functional consistencies of the identified cortical landmarks, we used working memory task-based fMRI data [12] to examine the results in Section 3.1. The working memory fMRI data provided 16 consistently activated brain regions, as shown by green boxes in Figs. 9a and 9b. By visual inspection, two cortical landmarks (red bubbles) extracted in Section 3.1 fall into the neighborhoods of two corresponding working memory regions (in yellow circles) consistently, as shown in Figs. 9a and 9b respectively. These close vicinities indicate that the locations of these two cortical landmarks identified by our approaches have consistent functional meanings in different brains, partly validating our methods.

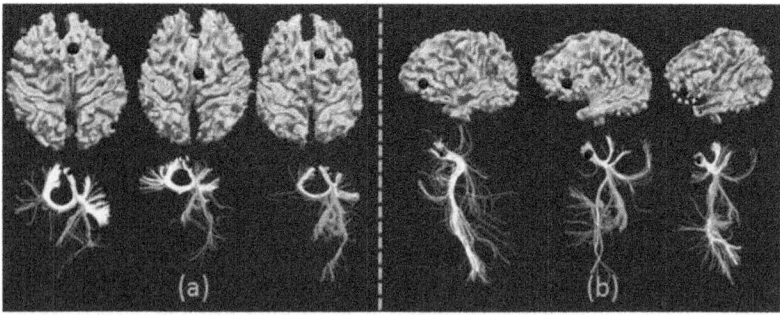

Fig. 9. Two examples of the spatial distribution of the working memory regions (green boxes) and one cortical landmark (red bubble) identified by our methods. Each column shows a subject. The yellow circles highlight the functional regions and the landmark. The second row shows the fibers connected to the landmarks. The cyan fibers are connections between the cortical landmark and subcortical regions, while the white fibers are connections between the cortical landmark and other cortical regions.

4 Conclusion

We presented a novel computational framework for identification of reliable cortical landmarks based on their structural connectivities to subcortical regions. In this framework, the subcortical regions serve as reference points for the definition of cortical connectional fingerprints. Then, 22 cortical regions with consistent cortico-subcortical connection patterns across subjects are selected as landmarks. Both qualitative and quantitative evaluations demonstrate the promise of this framework. In particular, a portion of the identified cortical landmarks were validated via task-based fMRI, which is widely accepted as a reliable approach to identifying corresponding functional regions across subjects. The work in this paper suggests that despite remarkable variation, there is deep-rooted regularity in the architecture of human brain, in particular, the regularity of cortico-subcortical connectivity patterns. Our future work will focus on in-depth analysis of the regularity and variability of the identified cortical landmarks in a larger scale dataset and further validation of the results via extensive task-based fMRI studies. In addition, the validated algorithmic pipeline will be applied to DTI datasets of brain diseases such as Alzheimer's disease for the purpose of elucidation of altered structural connectivities.

References

1. Passingham, R.E., et al.: The anatomical basis of functional localization in the cortex. Nat. Rev. Neurosci. 3(8), 606–616 (2002)
2. Young, M.P.: The organization of neural systems in the primate cerebral cortex. Proc. R. Soc. Lond, B. 252, 13–18 (1993)
3. Scannell, J.W., et al.: Analysis of connectivity in the cat cerebral cortex. J. Neurosci. 15, 1463–1483 (1995)
4. Behrens, T.E.J., et al.: Non-invasivemapping of connections between human thalamus and cortex using diffusion imaging. Nat. Neurosci. 6, 750–757 (2003)
5. Ashburner, J., et al.: Human Brain Function. Academic Press, London (2004)
6. Patenaude, B., Smith, S.M., Kennedy, D., Jenkinson, M.: A Bayesian Model of Shape and Appearance for Subcortical Brain NeuroImage (in press, 2011)
7. Liu, et al.: Reconstruction of Central Cortical Surface from MRI Brain Images: Method and Application. NeuroImage 40(3), 991–1002 (2007)
8. http://www.fmrib.ox.ac.uk/fsl/fdt/index.html
9. Liu, T., et al.: Brain tissue segmentation based on DTI data. Neuroimage 15: 38(1) (2007)
10. Patenaude, B., et al.: Improved surface models for FIRST. In: Human Brain Mapping Conference (2008)
11. Zöllei, L., et al.: Improved tractography alignment using combined volumetric and surface registration. Neuroimage 51(1), 206–213 (2010)
12. Faraco, C., Unsworth, N., Langley, J., Terry, D., Li, K., Zhang, D., Liu, T., Miller, S.: Complex span tasks and hippocampal recruitment during working memory. NeuroImage 55, 773–787 (2011)

T_1 Mapping, AIF and Pharmacokinetic Parameter Extraction from Dynamic Contrast Enhancement MRI Data

Gilad Liberman[1,3,4], Yoram Louzoun[2], Olivier Colliot[3], and Dafna Ben Bashat[4]

[1] Gonda Multidisciplinary Brain Research Center, Bar Ilan University,
Ramat Gan, Israel
[2] Department of Mathematics, Bar Ilan University, Ramat Gan, Israel
[3] Université Pierre et Marie Curie-Paris 6, CNRS UMR 7225, Inserm UMR S 975,
Centre de Recherche de l'Institut Cerveau-Moelle (CRICM), Paris, France
[4] Functional Brain center, The Wohl Institute for Advanced Imaging, Tel Aviv
Sourasky Medical Center, Tel Aviv, Israel

Abstract. Dynamic contrast enhanced (DCE) magnetic resonance imaging (MRI) is a sensitive, noninvasive technique for the assessment of microvascular properties of the tissue. Quantitative physiological parameters can be obtained using pharmacokinetic (PK) models that track contrast agents as it passes through the tissue vasculature. Such analysis usually requires prior knowledge of the voxels' T_1 values and of the Arterial Input Function (AIF). Therefore, relaxometry T_1 measurements are usually performed prior to contrast-agent injection and the AIF is manually or automatically extracted from the dynamic data. In this study, a method for a fully automatic analysis of DCE data for joint PK parameters, T_1 mapping and AIF extraction is proposed. Results are shown on simulated data compared to other methods and on data acquired from healthy subjects and patients with Glioblastoma who received anti-angiogenic therapy. The proposed method renders DCE analysis to be robust and easily applicable.

1 Introduction

Dynamic contrast enhancement (DCE) Magnetic resonance imaging (MRI) is a noninvasive method that provides vasculature information about the tissue. This method was shown to be sensitive and often used as indicator to monitor response to anti-angiogenic drugs in several organs including the brain [1]. In DCE, repeated T_1 weighted images are acquired with high temporal resolution, during the administration of a contrast agent resulting in a signal intensity time curve $S_v(t)$, at each voxel. This dynamic information shows the rate at which tissue enhances, and afterwards, the rate at which contrast agent washes out. The time curve can be converted into a contrast agent concentration time curve $C(t)$ and using a pharmacokinetic (PK) model, several physiological parameters can be extracted, such as vessels permeability, the volumes of the vessel and the extra-vascular extra-cellular space.

T. Liu et al. (Eds.): MBIA 2011, LNCS 7012, pp. 76–83, 2011.

In order to obtain the concentration time curve, a prior knowledge on the T_1 values within each voxel is needed. Therefore, a T_1 relaxometry experiment is performed prior to the DCE experiment. Inversion-recovery (IR) and saturation-recovery (SR) are the principal methods for T_1 measurements, yet their long acquisition times make them inapplicable for clinical use. Several alternative methods have been proposed for rapid and accurate measurement of the longitudinal relaxation time T_1. A commonly used method is the variable nutation angle method, that use a collection of spoiled gradient echo (SPGR) images over a range of flip angles. Although this method allows quick T_1 determination, it requires additional scanning and often suffers from B_1 inhomogeneity, and errors result from inaccurate flip angle.

Following this stage, the $C(t)$ is fitted to a PK model. Several PK models have been proposed including the general kinetic model, Patlak model and Tofts model [13]. This study used the extended Tofts-Kety model [9]. Most of the models require an auxiliary Arterial Input Function (AIF), which is $C(t)$ in the artery feeding the examined voxels. The AIF is artery, patient and scan dependent. Several studies suggest using common population average AIF such as the one provided by [7]. The AIF can also be approximated by averaging several $C(t)$s from voxels inside major arteries, which can be located manually or automatically. These approaches require that the scan time-resolution will be high enough for accurate AIF determination. Fit-based methods for extracting the AIF from $C(t)$s of multiple regions have been recently reported [5,12], where extraction of the AIF and PK parameters from the $C(t)$s are performed alternately using an expectation-maximization like algorithm, which is prone to local-minima problems. Yang [12] has noted the advantage of calculating the AIF at a higher time resolution than the scanning one, while Fluckiger [5] addressed the same problem by fitting the extracted AIF into a parametric formulation. We suggest a direct search over a parametric formulation of the AIF, thus less dependent on start point and local minimas.

While previously reported methods fitted the model to the $C(t)$, the algorithm proposed in this study fits the model and a T_1 value to the signal ratio to baseline curve. This enables us to extract the T_1 values from the DCE data itself, thus not requiring additional scan for T_1 mapping. Furthermore, using the signal ratio to baseline curve as a standard of reference enables a fair comparison between different algorithms, whereas comparison based on the $C(t)$ curves adds additional varables and necessitate additional calculation which depends on the analysis software / algorithm, and complicates comparison. The incorporation of the T_1 value into the fitting scheme renders the problem non-linear.

Several algorithms have been suggested for fitting of the $C(t)$ in order to extract PK parameters given the AIF. Murase [2] has formulated the differential equations of the extended Tofts-Kety model into simple matrix multiplication, resulting in a very efficient extraction of parameters. However this method implicitly assumes that the AIF can be approximated by its discrete low time-resolution form, and indeed was found in our study to be inaccurate, especially in sensitive areas such as those with low Signal-to-Noise Ratio (SNR), where the resulting inaccuracies are more pronounced. We propose a simple search over the non-linear term in the convolution formulation of the model. This enables the computation to be made in arbitrary time-resolution. We compare and evaluate our algorithm with Murase's as well as common non-linear curve-fitting techniques, including Simplex Simulated Annealing and Fletcher-Levenberg-Marquardt algorithm [4,3].

The following sections are organized as follows. Background and the proposed approach are presented in §2. The experiments and their results are discussed in §3 and the conclusions are given in §4.

2   Methods

2.1   Calculating the Signal Ratio to Baseline Curve

DCE MRI is usually acquired using a spoiled gradient echo (SPGR) sequence. The signal follows this equation [8]

$$S = M_0 \frac{(1 - E_1)\sin(\alpha)}{1 - E_1 \cos(\alpha)}. \tag{1}$$

where α is the flip angle, $E_1 = \exp(-TR/T_1)$ and M_0 includes the proton density, T_2 and T_2^* contributions and any fixed factor resulting from scanner settings. TR and FA are the repetition time and flip angle which are scan parameters and are fixed during the scan. The tissue's T_1 value is changing during the experiment as a function of the contrast agent concentration $C(t)$:

$$\Delta R_1(t) = R_1(t) - R_{10} = r_1 \cdot C(t). \tag{2}$$

where $R_{10} = 1/T_1$ is the relaxation rate at baseline (without contrast agent), $R_1(t)$ is the relaxation at time t and r_1 is the relaxivity coefficient of the contrast agent.

$$\Xi = \frac{S(t)}{S_0} = \frac{(1 - E_{10})(1 - E_1(t)\cos(\alpha))}{(1 - E_1(t))(1 - E_{10}\cos(\alpha))}. \tag{3}$$

Where $E_1(t) = \exp(-TR \cdot R_1(t))$. The baseline value S_0 can be computed by averaging the signal before contrast agent administration. The M_0 term includes a multiplicative $\exp(-TE/T_2^*)$ term. Although T_2^* changes in the presence of contrast agent, its effect on the signal is negligible due to the low TE values used in SPGR sequences.

2.2   Extraction of the PK Parameters and T_1 Values

Given T_1, $C(t)$ can be extracted from the signal ratio to baseline $\Xi(t)$ using equation (3). $C(t)$ can be modeled using the Extended Tofts-Kety model [9] by

$$\frac{d(C_t - v_p AIF_t)}{dt} = v_e k_{\text{ep}} AIF - k_{\text{ep}}(C_t - v_p AIF_t). \tag{4}$$

where AIF is the Arterial Input Function, the concentration of contrast agent in the feeding artery. The AIF is assumed to be the same for the whole analyzed volume of interest (VOI). k^{trans} and k_{ep} are the transfer rates between the blood plasma to the extra-vascular extra-cellular and back, respectively. v_e and v_p are the extra-vascular extra-cellular and the plasma relative volumes, respectively. The solution of the differential equation for $C(t)$ with initial conditions $AIF_0 = C_0 = 0$ was given by [9]

$$C(t) = k^{\text{trans}}(AIF(t) * \exp(-k_{\text{ep}}t)) + v_p AIF(t). \tag{5}$$

Where $*$ means convolution. The important pharmacokinetic parameter k^{trans} is equal to $v_e k_{\text{ep}}$. Following [2], integrating (4) leads to

$$C(t) = (k^{\text{trans}} + k_{\text{ep}}v_p) \int_0^t AIF(u)du - k_{\text{ep}} \int_0^t C(u)du + v_p AIF(t). \tag{6}$$

Discretizing, denote by $\overrightarrow{SAIF}$ and $\overrightarrow{SC}$ the cumulative sums of the AIF and the tissue contrast agent concentration curve, respectively, in the samples time points. The equation system resulting from (6) can thus be expressed in matrix form as

$$\overrightarrow{C} = (\overrightarrow{SAIF} \quad -\overrightarrow{SC} \quad \overrightarrow{AIF})\overrightarrow{X}^T. \tag{7}$$

$$\overrightarrow{X} = (k^{\text{trans}} + k_{\text{ep}}v_p \quad k_{\text{ep}} \quad v_p)$$

where vectors are columns and $\cdot^T$ means transpose. Given the AIF, X can be extracted by minimizing the least squares error and the PK parameters $k^{\text{trans}}, k_{\text{ep}}, v_e, v_p$ are approximated. Murase's method implicitly assumes that the AIF and the C_ts can be accurately approximated by the piecewise-linear curve induced by the data vectors. This might fail when the acquisition time-resolution is not high enough. Indeed, Murase's method was found to be inaccurate in our simulations and data for low SNR values. Therefore an alternative method, based on equation (5), is proposed in this study. Given the AIF and k_{ep}, the equation system can be formulated as

$$\overrightarrow{C} = (\overrightarrow{AIF * exp(k_{\text{ep}}u)} \quad \overrightarrow{AIF})\overrightarrow{Y}^T. \tag{8}$$

$$\overrightarrow{Y} = (k^{\text{trans}} \quad v_p)$$

and solved similarly. The solution was compared to the solution given while fixing either k^{trans} or v_p for their minimal and maximal values, and the one with minimal error was selected. Finding the correct k_{ep} is found by exhaustive search, i.e. repeating the process for several values of k_{ep} (21 values, spaced non-uniformly in $[0, \frac{\max k^{\text{trans}}}{\min v_e} = \frac{2.2}{0.15} = 14.667]\text{min}^{-1}$).

We suggest finding T_1 by fitting to the signal ratio to baseline curve $\varXi$ using exhaustive search in biological range (22 values spaced uniformly in $[300, 4000]\text{ms}$). For each T_1 value, C_t is calculated from $\varXi$ using eq. (3) and the PK parameters are extracted using (7) (during computationally extensive

AIF search) or (8) (given final AIF). Using the PK parameters and T_1, we simulate the signal ratio to baseline curve $\hat{\Xi}$ and compare it to Ξ using the Euclidean norm. Added penalty on improbable T_1 values can be used at this level, corresponding, in a Bayesian interpretation, to prior on the expected T_1 in the voxel, which can result from relaxometry or segmentation. The simulation is done using equation (5) and requires convolution. Both the AIF and $exp(k_{ep}t)$ can be calculated for arbitrary time points, and this convolution is calculated numerically in higher time resolution to increase accuracy.

We compare the results obtained using the proposed method with Murase's method, a conventional fitting method [3] and a fast simulated annealing variant [4]. For estimating the inaccuracies resulting from fit-based T_1 approximation, results are compared based on simulated data with the parameters estimated by the mentioned methods with given true T_1 values.

2.3 AIF Extraction

Parker [7] has suggested to model the AIF using two Gaussians and a sigmoid which correspond to the main and second cycle contrast agent boluses and the washout:

$$AIF = \sum_{i=1}^{2} A_i N(\tau_i, \sigma_i) + \frac{\alpha \exp(-\beta t)}{(1 + \exp(-s(t - \tau_0)))}. \tag{9}$$

Where N is the normal distribution. Mean values for the model parameters were also given. (9) can be modified to yield a version more fitted for function search by using relative values for the amplitudes (A_2, α relative to A_1) and times (τ_2, τ_0 relative to τ_1). We denote by $AIFf()$ the AIF model given by the modified version of (9).

The proposed cost function is the maximum over the sum square error for the given signal ratio to baseline curve, normalized by its maximum minus one, i.e. its maximal relative enhancement value.

$$\arg\min_{\theta} \max_{i \in Clusters} \frac{\|\hat{\Xi}_{i\,AIFf(\theta)} - \Xi_i\|^2}{\max_j \Xi_i(j) - 1}. \tag{10}$$

On real data, the curves used are the result of a cluster analysis over all of the brain's voxels (healthy subjects) or a large VOI around the lesion (patients). The VOI is masked by the following criteria - Minimal enhancement of 2%, a signal over a specific threshold value (experimental defined) and probability of being a gray or white matter tissue more than 30% (as defined using SPM's segmentation module [11]). The cluster analysis used is Expectation-Maximization (EM) over Mixture of Gaussians (MoG) model [6] with 100 clusters. The clustering is calculated over the voxels' signal curves (rather than the signal ratio to baseline curve). The bolus starting point is approximated in a competitive manner by clustering the medians of the signals of all the brain volume at each time point into 3 clusters and selecting the first value which is classified into a cluster different than that of the first time point. Voxels for which the maximal enhancement occurs more than one acquisition before the approximated bolus starting point are masked out. The search was done by running SIMPSA [4] twice. The first run uses the parameters given by Parker [7] as a starting point and works on a reduced set of data for acceleration. In a second step, more clusters are used, and the result of the first run is the starting point. Up to 5 clusters are automatically chosen for the first SIMPSA run by selecting the clusters with the highest maximal signal to baseline ratio, while assuring that at least 2 clusters with visible contribution of the plasma to $C(t)$ are selected. For the second run, 40 clusters are randomly chosen. Clusters with noisy curve are discarded.

3   Experiments and Results

Simulated Data. To test the extraction of the PK parameters, 500 signal ratio to baseline curves were simulated using the AIF given at [7], with T_1 and PK parameters selected randomly in biological ranges (T_1 in $[300, 4000]$ ms, k^{trans} in $[0, 2.2]$ min^{-1}, v_e in $[0.15, 1]$, v_p in $[0, 0.3]$). Mean Absolute Relative Difference (ARD) was used as the statistical criteria.

Results of the simulated data, obtained using the proposed method compared to SIMPSA, FLM and Murase's method, are reported in Table 1. Note that the proposed method yield the smaller ARD values for all parameters with and without prior knowledge of T_1 values, compared to the other methods.

For AIF extraction tests, 100 runs were done with the AIF model of eq. (9) on randomly selected parameters around the ones given in [7] (between half and double the reported value, except for τ_1, between 0.8 to 3 times the reported value). Additionally, a small amount of noise on the AIF model parameters was added to each simulated voxel (Multiplicative factor of $N(1, 0.05)$) to simulate the changes in AIF between feeding artery in the VOI. Finally, an additive Gaussian noise ($\sigma = 0.08$) was added to the simulated signal ratio time curve to simulate noise in acquisition. This noise amplitude was extracted by the std. of the signal before contrast agent administration for a representative patient. We used $r_1 = 1$. This value gave maximal signal ratio curve values similar to ones observed in real data (around 6).

Results are reported in Table 2. The proposed method using SIMPSA yielded the smallest ARD values for the PK parameters, excluding k_{ep}.

Table 1. Comparison of mean ARD values for the PK parameters. The last 3 columns show results when T_1 was assumed to be known. For Murase's method, the T_1 value was found using the same exhaustive search as in the proposed method.

Method	k^{trans}	v_e	v_p	T_1	k^{trans}	v_e	v_p
SIMPSA	2.66	0.82	1.66	**0.42**	1.54	0.56	0.72
FLM	2.73	0.71	0.70	0.52	1.57	0.91	0.74
Murase	0.94	1.08	1.09	0.45	0.30	0.50	0.46
Proposed method	**0.67**	**0.54**	**0.57**	**0.42**	**0.22**	**0.12**	**0.16**

Table 2. Comparison of mean ARD values for the PK parameters, after AIF estimation using only clusters with strong enhancement, using all data or in two steps

PK Method	AIF Method	k^{trans}	v_e	v_p	T_1	k_{ep}
Murase	SIMPSA	0.93	1.50	0.68	0.52	0.50
Murase	SIMPSA, full data	1.02	1.91	0.69	0.59	0.59
Murase	SIMPSA, 2 steps	1.00	1.80	0.70	0.58	0.59
Proposed method	SIMPSA	0.75	0.83	0.54	0.55	0.52
Proposed method	SIMPSA, full data	0.88	1.11	0.57	0.59	0.61
Proposed method	SIMPSA, 2 steps	0.97	1.08	0.59	0.60	0.67

MRI Data. The proposed algorithm was tested on real MRI data obtained from five healthy controls and five longitudinal studies of two patients with progressive recurrent glioblastoma along the administration of an anti-angiogenic therapy (Bevacizumab) combined with Irinotecan. The signal ratio to baseline curves were fitted accurately for all studies. For the control group, the different vascular regions are clearly visible (see Fig. 1 top). A representative result for a longitudinal study of a patient with Glioblastoma is shown in Fig. 1 left. As expected, after two weeks of anti-angiogenic therapy, a reduction of k^{trans} and v_p is visible in the tumor area.

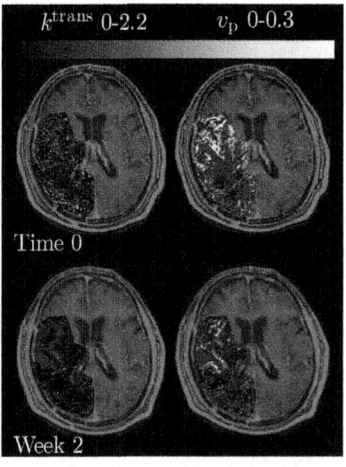

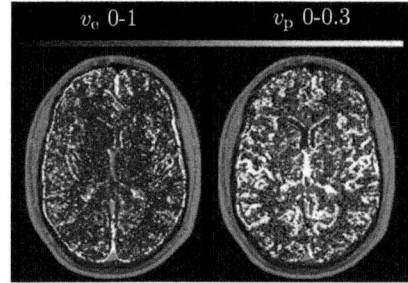

Fig. 1. Left: k^{trans} and v_p (columns) maps for a longitudinal study of a patient with GBM. Weeks 0, 2 (rows) of anti-angiogenic treatment. Top: v_e and v_p maps for a healthy subject, showing vascular regions.

4   Conclusion

This work proposes a method for PK parameters extraction by curve fitting to the DCE data. The choice of fitting to the actual DCE data rather than concentration time curves approximated using pre-computed T_1 values renders the method more applicable to acquired data and independent of relaxometry calculation. The automatic identification of the AIF renders the method fully automatic. The pseudo-sampling during calculation enables the system to maintain accuracy while retaining high efficacy through matrix operations. The method has been applied to both simulated and real data resulting in good results. Future work will incorporate optimizing global parameters such as the flip angle.

Acknowledgments and Funding. This work was supported by the James S. McDonnell Foundation number 220020176. We are grateful to the patients and their families, who so willingly participated in this study and to Vicki Meiers for editorial assistance.

References

1. O'Connor, J.P.B., Jackson, A., Parker, G.J.M., Jayson, G.C.: DCE-MRI biomarkers in the clinical evaluation of antiangiogenic and vascular disrupting agents. Brit. J. Can. 96, 189–195 (2007)
2. Murase, K.: Efficient method for calculating kinetic parameters using T1-weighted dynamic contrast-enhanced magnetic resonance imaging. Mag. Res. Med. 51, 858–862 (2004)
3. Fletcher, R.: A modified Marquardt subroutine for nonlinear least squares. Atom. Res. Est. AERE-R6799 (1971)
4. Cardoso, M.F., Salcedo, R., Feyo de Azevedo, S.: The simplex-simulated annealing approach to continuous non-linear optimization. Comp. Chem. Eng. 20, 1065–1080 (1996)
5. Fluckiger, J.U., Schabel, M.C., DiBella, E.V.R.: Model-based blind estimation of kinetic parameters in dynamic contrast enhanced (DCE)-MRI. Mag. Res. Med. 62, 1477–1486 (2009)
6. Bouman, C. A., Shapiro, M., Cook, G. W., Atkins, C. B., Cheng, H.: Cluster: An unsupervised algorithm for modeling gaussian mixtures, https://engineering.purdue.edu/~bouman/
7. Parker, G.J., Roberts, C., Macdonald, A., Buonaccorsi, G.A., Cheung, S., Buckley, D.L., Jackson, A., Watson, Y., Davies, K., Jayson, G.C.: Experimentally-derived functional form for a population-averaged high-temporal-resolution arterial input function for dynamic contrast-enhanced MRI. Mag. Res. Med. 56, 993–1000 (2006)
8. Deoni, S.C., Rutt, B.K., Peters, T.M.: Rapid combined T1 and T2 mapping using gradient recalled acquisition in the steady state. Mag. Res. Med. 49, 515–526 (2003)
9. Tofts, P.S., Kermode, A.G.: Measurement of the blood-brain barrier permeability and leakage space using dynamic MR imaging. 1. Fundamental concepts. Mag. Res. Med. 17, 357–367 (1991)
10. Tofts, P.S., Brix, G., Buckley, D.L., Evelhoch, J.L., Henderson, E., Knopp, M.V., Larsson, H.B., Lee, T.-Y., Mayr, N.A., Parker, G.J., Port, R.E., Taylor, J., Weisskoff, R.M.: Estimating kinetic parameters from dynamic contrast-enhanced t1-weighted MRI of a diffusable tracer: Standardized quantities and symbols. J. Mag. Res. Imag. 10, 223–232 (1999)
11. Ashburner, J., Friston, K.J.: Unied segmentation. NeuroImage 26, 839–851 (2005)
12. Yang, C., Karczmar, G.S., Medved, M., Stadler, W.M.: Multiple reference tissue method for contrast agent arterial input function estimation. Mag. Res. Med. 58, 1266–1275 (2007)
13. Srikanchana, R., Thomasson, D., Choyke, P., Dwyer, A.: A Comparison of Pharmacokinetic Models of Dynamic Contrast Enhanced MRI. In: 17th IEEE Symposium on Computer-Based Medical Systems, p. 361. IEEE Computer Society, Los Alamitos (2004)

Ventricle Shape Analysis for Centenarians, Elderly Subjects, MCI and AD Patients

Zhaojin Gong[1], Jianfeng Lu[1], Jia Chen[1], Yaping Wang[2,3], Yixuan Yuan[2], Tuo Zhang[2], Lei Guo[2], L Stephen Miller[4], and the Georgia Centenarian Study*

[1] School of Computer Science, Nanjing Univ. of Science and Technology, Nanjing, China
{Zhaojingong,xiaosa2356}@126.com, lujf@mail.njust.edu.cn
[2] School of Automation, Northwestern Polytechnical Univ., Xi'an China
{yaping.wang333,yuanyixuan817,zhangtuo.npu,guolei.npu}@gmail.com
[3] Department of Radiology, UNC Chapel Hill, USA
[4] Department of Psychology and Bioimaging Research Center, Univ. of Georgia, Athens, GA
lsmiller@uga.edu

Abstract. In this paper, we examined the ventricle shapes of centenarian brains in comparison with those of elderly, mild cognitive impairment (MCI) and Alzheimer's Disease (AD). The MRI datasets obtained from Centenarian Study (CS) and the ADNI project are analyzed via the spherical harmonics (SPHARM) shape analysis pipeline. Our results indicate that if the elderly brains are used as comparison baseline, there is no significant difference between centenarian and elderly brains, while the differences between elderly and MCI/AD brains are significant; if the centenarian brains are used as comparison baseline, the differences between centenarian and MCI brains are moderate, but much more significant differences between AD and centenarian brains appear. Further comparisons of volume and shape analysis suggest that ventricle shape characteristics could potentially be a more sensitive biomarker of AD progression than the traditionally assumed ventricle volumes.

Keywords: MRI, shape analysis, AD, MCI, centenarian.

1 Introduction

Ventricle enlargement has been conceived as a marker of a variety of brain diseases such as Alzheimer's disease [8]. Hence, quantitative measurement of ventricle volume based on cross-sectional or longitudinal MRI data has been of keen interest in the brain imaging community [6, 10]. While volume measurement is a natural choice in many applications for ventricle analysis, shape measurement provides additional information about structural changes such as bending or flattening of ventricle in a focused location. For instance, the thickening of the occipital horn of the ventricles may not be reflected in the overall volumetric measurement [10].

In this paper, we examined the ventricle shapes of the centenarian brains based on the MRI data acquired during CS. The CS database has biological, psychological, and social data that are pertinent to the survival and functioning of the population of 244

T. Liu et al. (Eds.): MBIA 2011, LNCS 7012, pp. 84–92, 2011.

centenarians and 80 matched 80-90 year old controls [11]. Then, we employed the SPHARM shape analysis pipeline described in [10] for ventricle shape analysis. The main advantage of SPHARM is that it is hierarchical, global, and multi-scale. This pipeline has been reported to have good performance in brain structure shape analysis [6]. Our results on the CS and ADNI MRI datasets demonstrate that centenarian brains are similar to the elderly aging group in terms of their ventricle shapes, but have moderate and significant differences compared with MCI and AD brains respectively. The major contribution of this paper is that we design and apply an algorithmic pipeline on a unique centenarian dataset and reported interesting results.

2   Method

2.1   Overview

Fig.1 shows the flowchart of our processing and analysis pipeline. The processing and analysis steps are as follows: (1) Registration of MRI images. All of the raw MRI images in both CS and ADNI datasets are registered to a template space in order to remove global variations. (2) Ventricle segmentation using 3D snakes. All of the ventricle shapes are reconstructed. (3) The left and right ventricles are analyzed separately. (4) Shape description

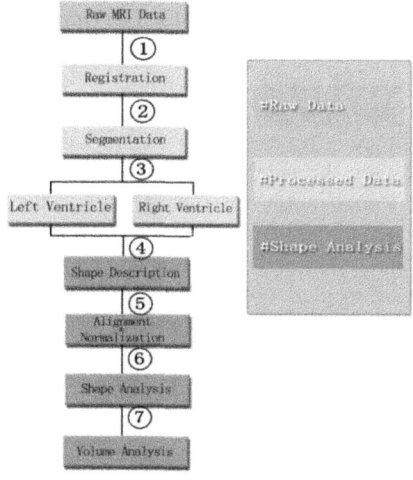

Fig. 1. The flowchart of the analysis pipeline

using SPHARM. In this step, all of the ventricle shape meshes are represented by the SPHARM. (5) Shape alignment and normalization. The shape alignment and normalization modules in the SPHARM software package [10] are applied to process the ventricle shape further. (6) Local testing of group differences using the Hotelling T^2 metric. The statistical shape difference is analyzed. (7) Volume analysis. The ventricle volumes from the CS and ADNI datasets are quantitatively analyzed in addition to shape analysis.

2.2   Materials and Pre-processing

Two MRI datasets are used for the ventricle shape comparison. The first dataset includes 26 CS subjects. The MRI data was acquired post-mortem on a 3T GE MRI scanner. The resolution of CS structural MRI T1 data is 1mm*1mm*1mm. In additional to the CS MRI data, the ADNI dataset [11] that includes elderly, MCI and AD patients is also used for comparison. Subjects that are between 70 and 80 years old are randomly selected from the ADNI dataset for the comparison study. Totally, 15 AD, 28 MCI, and 22 normal samples are used in this paper.

Then, a template image is randomly selected from an elderly subject in the ADNI dataset, and all of other MRI images are warped to this template space via the FSL FLIRT linear registration tool. It is expected that this step will facilitate the following steps of shape analysis by removing global variation of the sizes and shapes of the ventricles. After image registration, we then use a deformable model based on the 3D snake algorithm [1] to extract the ventricles from the MRI images. First, considering that the ventricle is cerebralspinal fluid (CSF) with significantly lower T1 image intensity, an image intensity threshold is empirically set to roughly segment the ventricle, and then the segmented shapes are selected as the initialization for the 3D snake algorithm. Then, the deformable model [1] was deformed to the ventricle boundaries as shown in Fig.2. All segmented ventricles were visually verified by experts for quality control.

2.3   SPHARM Methods

2.3.1   SPHARM
It is well-known that the associated Legendre polynomials are orthogonal, and orthonormal basis functions can express any piecewise continuous function over [-1, 1] as a linear combination of an infinite series of linearly independent basis functions [9]. Then, the associated Legendre polynomial definition is:

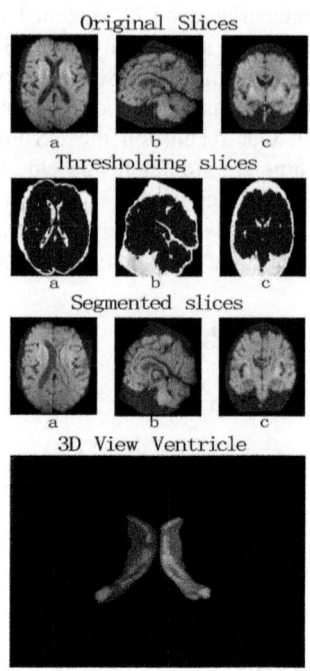

Fig. 2. The process of extracting the ventricle. The top row shows the original image slices, the second row is the result after applying the threshold, the third row presents the segmented ventricles, and the last row is the 3D view of the ventricle shape

$$p_l^m = \frac{(-1)^m}{2^l l!} \sqrt{(1-x^2)^m} \frac{d^{l+m}}{dx^{l+m}} (x^2-1)^l \tag{1}$$

where the two integer arguments l and m are constrained by $l \in N_0$ and $m \in [0, l]$. Here, l is used as the band index to divide the class into bands of functions resulting in a total of $(l+1)l$ polynomials for l-th band series. In the representation of spherical harmonics, the spherical polar coordinate system (Fig. 3) is used. The spherical polar coordinate system is defined by two angles θ and ϕ, where $0 \le \phi < 2\pi$ describes the azimuthal angle in the xy-plane originating at the x-axis and $0 \le \theta < \pi$ denotes the polar angle from the z-axis (Fig.3).

Then, the spherical polar coordinates is used to express the circularly symmetric function, which is independent of ϕ, in terms of the associated Legendre polynomial by mapping θ into the [-1, 1] by using $\cos\theta$. In order to ensure the orthogonality in case of non-circular symmetric functions, it can be realized by combining the associated Legendre polynomials for the θ dependence with the sine and cosine functions for the ϕ dependent part. Therefore, the definition of the complex-valued spherical harmonic series with two arguments $l \in N_0$ and $-l \le m \le l$ is given by:

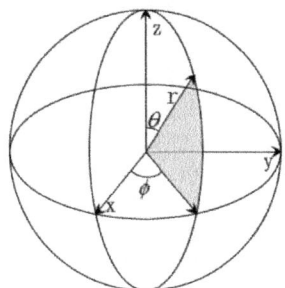

Fig. 3. Spherical polar coordinate system

$$Y_l^m(\theta,\phi) = N_l^{|m|} p_l^{|m|}(\cos\theta)e^{im\phi} \tag{2}$$

where N_l^m denotes a normalization coefficient, and N_l^m is derived as follows:

$$N_l^m = \sqrt{\frac{2l+1}{4\pi}\frac{(l-m)!}{(l+m)!}} \tag{3}$$

where the l in Legendre polynomials denotes the band index. And $e^{im\phi}$ is the Euler identity and its definition is as follows:

$$e^{im\phi} = \cos(m\phi)+i\sin(m\phi) \tag{4}$$

Afterwards, the spherical harmonic basis is used to express the surface of the ventricle as follows.

$$surf(\theta,\phi) = \sum_{l=0}^{\infty}\sum_{m=-l}^{l}c_l^m Y_l^m(\theta,\phi) \tag{5}$$

where $surf(\theta,\phi)$ denotes the surface of the ventricle. The coefficients c_l^m are numeric solution which is solved by the Monte Carlo estimator [3] and can be expressed as follows:

$$c_l^m = \frac{1}{n}\sum_j^n f(x_j)y_l^m(x_j)w(x_j) \tag{6}$$

where $w(x_j)$ is a weighting function with value of $1/4\pi$, accounting for an equal distribution of samples on the surface of a unit sphere. l represents the different scale to express the ventricle (Fig. 4).

2.3.2   Point Distribution Model (PDM) Based on SPHARM

Based on the SPHARM representation of ventricle surfaces in the above section, the spherical parameters are sampled uniformly on the spheres for statistical analysis. It is noted that the equidistant sampling on a sphere will lead to a dense sampling around the two poles ($\theta = 0, \theta = \pi$) and a coarse sampling around the equator ($\theta = \pi/2$) [10]. In order to obtain well-distributed points, we subdivide linear and uniform icosahedrons, thus a good approximation of a homogeneous sampling on the spherical parameter space and the object space can be achieved [10]. The subdivision is linear in the number of subdivisions along each edge of the original icosahedrons, rather than the recursive subdivisions [6]. Locations (θ_i, ϕ_i) of the subdivided icosahedrons could be pre-calculated, and then the PDM is directly calculated from the coefficients [10]. The sampled point x_i at the location (θ_i, ϕ_i) is obtained from the Eq. (7), where K is a constant:

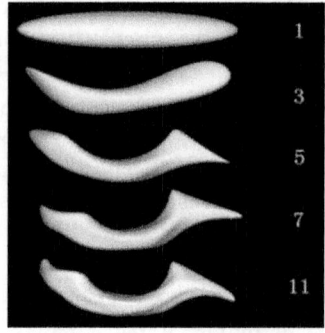

Fig. 4. SPHARM shape description of the ventricle at different scales (1, 3, 5, 7, and 11 respectively)

$$x_i = \sum_{l=0}^{K} \sum_{m=-l}^{l} c_l^m Y_l^m(\theta_i, \phi_i) \tag{7}$$

In this paper, the subdivision level is set to 10 which can represent the ventricle shape quite well based on our extensive observations.

2.3.3   Alignment and Normalization

Alignment and normalization are prerequisite steps for calculating the similarity and difference between shapes. Before alignment and normalization, the correspondence between subjects is achieved by normalizing the parameters to one template using the first order of SPHARM (see Fig.4). The normalization is then achieved by rotation of the parameterization, such that the spherical equator, $0°$ and $90°$ longitudes coincide with those of the first order ellipsoids. After this processing, correspondences between surface points across different shapes are established [6].

For shape analysis study, there are two methods: no scaling normalization and scaling inversely to the intra-cranial cavity volume (ICV). In this paper, the rigid-body Procrustes alignment [4] is followed by scaling inversely to the ICV. The original scale analysis is an unbiased raw analysis, whereas the ICV scaling considers the differences in aging, head size and etc, and can approximately normalize gender and age differences. After the above steps of shape description, correspondence establishment, alignment and scaling normalization, the next step in the shape analysis is to examine the differences between groups at each surface location. We use the Hotelling T^2 as a difference metric of two groups. The null hypothesis is that the distribution of the locations at each spatial element is the same for each subject regardless of group. Permutations among the two groups satisfy the exchangeability condition, i.e., they leave the distribution of the statistic of interest unaltered under the null hypothesis. Given the first group S_i with n_1 members, $i = 1,2,...,n_1$ and the second group $S_i^{'}$ with n_2 members, $i = 1,2,...,n_2$, $M \leq \binom{n_1 + n_2}{n_1}$ permutation samples are created. The value of M from 20000 and up should yield results that are negligibly different from using all permutations [7].

3   Results

In this section, we present how to apply the SPHARM algorithm pipeline to the ventricles analysis of AD, MCI, normal subjects, and centenarians. In this study, we used 15 AD, 28 MCI, 26 centenarian and 22 normal samples.

3.1   Results of Using Normal Brain as the Baseline

Fig. 5 and Fig. 6 show the results of comparison using the normal brain as the baseline. It is apparent that there are significant differences between the normal aging group and MCI/AD groups, for both the left and right ventricles. This result is reasonable, given the neuropathological processes in the MCI and AD progression.

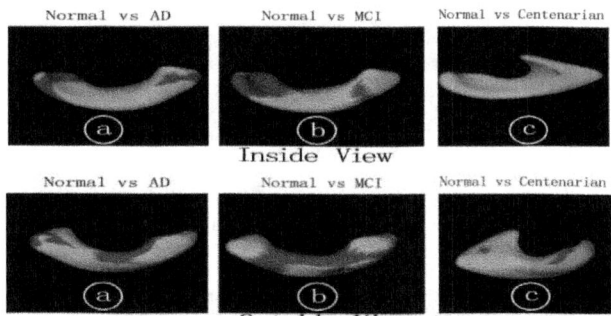

Fig. 5. The inside and outside views of comparison results for the left ventricles with the normal aging group as the baseline.Red and green stand for significant and non-significant respectively.

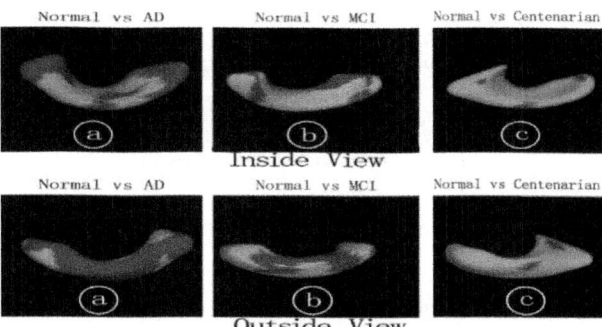

Fig. 6. The inside and outside views of comparison result for the right ventricles with the normal group as the baseline. Red and green stand for significant and non-significant.

However, the difference between the centenarian group and normal aging group is minor. This result suggests that the ventricle shapes of centenarian brains are similar to the elderly aging group. It is interesting that the difference between the normal aging group and the AD group is more on the right ventricle than that on the left ventricle, as shown in the left columns in Fig. 5 and Fig. 6.

3.2   Results of Using Centenarian Brains as the Baseline

Fig.7 and Fig. 8 show the results of comparison results by using the centenarian brains as the baseline. The results for the centenarian and normal aging brains are the same as those in Fig. 5 and Fig. 6. Here, the difference between the centenarian and MCI brain is minor, as shown in the middle columns of Fig. 7 and Fig. 8. However, the difference between the AD and centenarian brains is significant, as shown in the first columns in Fig. 7 and Fig. 8.

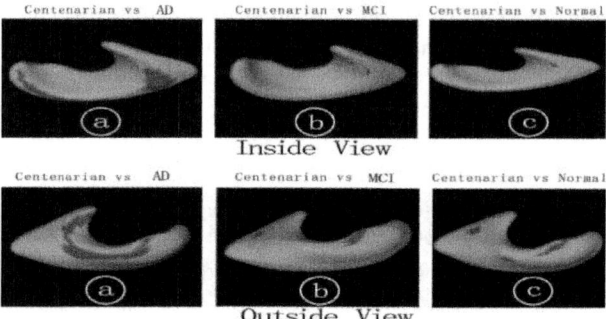

Fig. 7. The inside and outside views of comparison results for the left ventricles with the centenarian group as the baseline. Red and green stand for significant and non-significant.

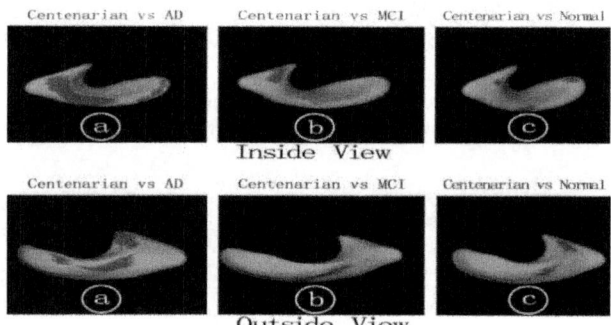

Fig. 8. The inside and outside views of results for the right ventricles with the centenarian group as the baseline. Red and green stand for significant and non-significant.

3.3   Volume Analysis Results

In addition to the shape analysis, we performed volume analysis as well. The volume distributions of the left and right ventricles for the AD, MCI, centenarian and normal

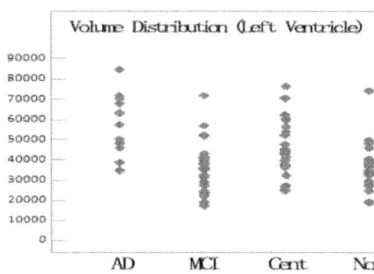 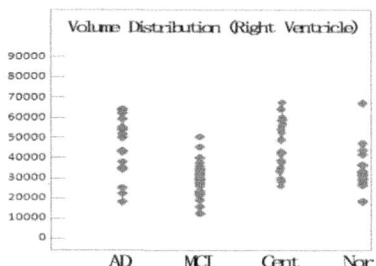

Fig. 9. Volume distributions of left (left) and right (right) ventricles for the four subject groups. Here, Cent and Nor stand for centenarian and normal aging brains respectively.

aging brains are shown in Fig.9. It can be seen that for the left ventricle, the AD group has the largest volumes, while the normal aging group has the smallest ventricles. The centenarian brains are between AD and MCI groups. For the right ventricle, the centernaran brains have the largest volumes, even larger than the AD group. It is interesting that the MCI group has the smallest volumes. However, as shown in Sections 3.1 and 3.2, the ventricle shapes of centenarian brains are quite similar to normal aging brain. Therefore, the results of shape and volume analysis in Sections 3.1-3.3 suggest that the shape difference might be a more sensitive marker of AD progression than the traditionally assumed ventricle volumes.

4   Conclusion and Discussion

We performed shape and volume analysis of ventricles of elderly aging, centenarian, MCI and AD subjects via the SPHARM algorithm pipeline. Our main result indicates that the centenarian brains' ventricles have relatively large volumes, but their shapes are similar to those in the aging brains. This result might suggest that ventricle shape characteristics could potentially be a more sensitive biomarker of AD progression than the traditionally assumed ventricle volumes [8].

It should be noted that the centenarian MRI data is postmortem. It is possible that the loss of CSF and postmortem MRI scan preparation could cause ventricle shape deformation. However, we believe that these deformations will not cause significant influence on the shape analysis results, as the global registration in section 2.2 and the shape alignment in section 2.3.3 can account for those deformations to some extent. In addition, the postmortem preparations for different centenarian subjects were separate and should not cause systematic errors to the segmented ventricle volumes and reconstructed shapes. The volume analysis in section 3.3 could underestimate the volumes of centenarian brains due to the loss of CSF fluid in postmortem brains. Even though the centenarian ventricle volumes were underestimated, we can still have the conclusion that the centenarian brains ventricles have relatively large volumes, but their shapes are similar to those in the elderly aging brains. Hence, the underestimation of ventricle volumes in centenarian brains will strengthen our conclusion, instead of weakening our conclusion.

Acknowledgements. This work is funded by the QingLan Project and Priority Academic Program Development of Jiangsu Higher Education Institutions.

References

1. Xu, C.Y., Prince, J.L.: Snakes, Shapes, and Gradient Vector Flow. IEEE Trans. Image Processing 7(3) (March 1998)
2. Kelemen, A., Szekely, G., Gerig, G.: Elastic model-based segmentation of 3D neuroradiological data sets. IEEE Trans. Med. Imaging 18 (1999)
3. Hammersley, J.M., Handscomb, D.C.: Monte Carlo Methods. Methuen & Co Ltd., London (1964)
4. Bookstein, F.L.: Morphometric Tools for Landmark Data: Geometry and Biology. Cambridge University Press, Cambridge (1991)
5. Seber, G.A.F.: Multivariate Observations. John Wiley & Sons, Chichester (1984)
6. Styner, M., Oguz, I.: Framework for the Statistical Shape Analysis of Brain Structures using SPHARM-PDM. In: The Insight Journal - 2006 MICCAI Open Science Workshop (2006)
7. Edgington, E.S. (ed.): Randomization Tests. Academic Press, London (1995)
8. Nestor, S., et al.: Changes in brain ventricle volume associated, with mild cognitive impairment and alzheimer disease in subjects participating in the alzheimer's disease neuroimaging initiative. Alzheimer's and Dementia (2007)
9. Schönefeld, V.: Spherical Harmonics, http://heim.c-otto.de/~volker/prosem_paper.pdf
10. Gerig, G., et al.: Shape analysis of brain ventricles using spharm. In: CVPR Mathematical Methods in Biomedical Image Analysis, pp. 171–178 (2001)
11. Jessica, D.: Alzheimer's Disease Neuroimaging Initiative Improve Power of Future Studies. Neurology Reviews 17(7), 13 (2007)

Accurate and Consistent 4D Segmentation of Serial Infant Brain MR Images

Li Wang[1], Feng Shi[1], Pew-Thian Yap[1], John H.Gilmore[2], Weili Lin[3], and Dinggang Shen[1],*

[1] IDEA Lab, Department of Radiology and BRIC
dgshen@med.unc.edu
[2] Department of Psychiatry,
[3] MRI Lab, Department of Radiology and BRIC
University of North Carolina at Chapel Hill, USA

Abstract. Accurate and consistent segmentation of infant brain MR images plays an important role in quantifying the early brain development, especially in longitudinal studies. However, due to rapid maturation and myelination of brain tissues in the first year of life, white-gray matter contrast undergoes dramatic changes. In fact, the contrast inverses around 6 months of age, where the white and gray matter tissues are isointense and hence exhibit the lowest contrast, posing significant challenges for segmentation algorithms. In this paper, we propose a novel longitudinally guided level set method for segmentation of serial infant brain MR images, acquired from 2 weeks up to 1.5 years of age. The proposed method makes optimal use of T1, T2 and the diffusion weighted images for complimentary tissue distribution information to address the difficulty caused by the low contrast. A longitudinally consistent term, which constrains the distance across the serial images within a biologically reasonable range, is employed to obtain temporally consistent segmentation results. The proposed method has been applied on 22 longitudinal infant subjects with promising results.

1 Introduction

The first year of life is the most dynamic phase of postnatal brain development. The brain undergoes rapid tissue growth and experiences development of a wide range of cognitive and motor functions. For precise quantification of structural growth, algorithms dedicated to accurate tissue segmentation of infant brains in the first year of life is indispensable. Current methods are able to segment neonates (less than 3 months) and infants (over 1-year-old) with great success [1]. However, works dealing with the segmentation of serial infant images in the first years of life have been few. During this period of growth, the contrast between white matter (WM) and gray matter (GM) reverses owing to maturation and myelination. There are three distinct WM/GM contrast patterns in images of developmentally normal infants (in chronological order) [2]: infantile (birth),

---

* Corresponding author.

T. Liu et al. (Eds.): MBIA 2011, LNCS 7012, pp. 93–101, 2011.

isointense, and adult-like (10 months onward). As an illustration, we show in Fig. 1 a series of longitudinal MR images for an infant scanned every 3 months, starting from the second week. From the T1 images, it can be seen that the intensity of WM is initially lower than that of GM, but becomes gradually brighter, resulting in a contrast pattern that resembles adults. The opposite trend can be observed for T2 images. At around 6 months of age, the WM and GM exhibit almost the same intensity level (see the third column of Fig. 1), resulting in the lowest WM/GM contrast and great difficulties for segmentation. Few studies have addressed the tissue segmentation on isointense stage infants, and the attempts are also hindered by the insufficient contrast T1/T2 image provided, especially at the subcortical regions. In addition, those voxel-wise methods [1,3] cannot provide smooth and closed cortical surface as the final segmentation outcome and are also unable to guarantee the consistency of results across the serial infant images.

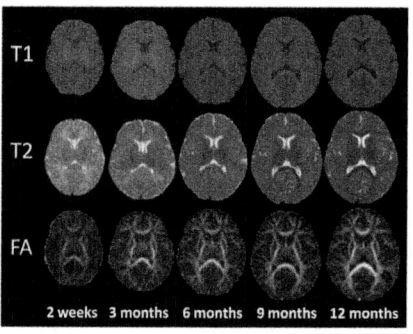

Fig. 1. T1, T2 and FA images of an infant scanned at 2 weeks, 3, 6, 9 and 12 months

The fractional anisotropy (FA) images from diffusion tensor imaging (DTI) (last row of Fig. 1) provide rich information of major fiber bundles, especially in the subcortical regions where GM and WM are hardly distinguishable in the T1/T2 images. Notably, the WM structure remains very consistent throughout all time points, proving partly the notion that the majority of the fibers exist at birth. In this work, we employ complementary information from multiple modalities by using T1, T2 and FA images to deal with the problem of insufficient tissue contrast. Information from these images are fed into a novel longitudinally guided level-set-based framework for consistent segmentation of the serial infant images. To introduce temporally consistent segmentation results, we enforce a longitudinal constraint term that is in accordance to the fact that global brain structures of the same full-term infant remain similar at different developmental stages [4]. Specifically, the distance between the tissue boundaries of the serial images are kept within a biologically reasonable range. The proposed method, tested on 22 subjects, shows promising results.

2   Method

The proposed method utilizes the multi-modality statistical information, cortical thickness constraint, and longitudinal constraint to derive an accurate and consistent segmentation of serial infant brain MR images. In the following subsections, we will discuss the formulation of the proposed energy.

2.1   Multi-modality Data Fitting Term

To robustly segment each time-point image, we make optimal use of T1, T2 and FA images. $t = \{0, 3, 6, ...\}$ denotes the age of infant scan, and index $j \in \{T1, T2, FA\}$ denotes the modality, i.e., T1, T2 and FA, respectively. Therefore, $I_{t,T1}$, $I_{t,T2}$, and $I_{t,FA}$ denote the T1, T2 and FA images at time-point t. Letting $\Phi_t = (\phi_{1,t}, \phi_{2,t}, \phi_{3,t})$ and by using Heaviside function H, three level set functions[1] $\phi_{1,t}$, $\phi_{2,t}$ and $\phi_{3,t}$ are employed to define regions $M_i(\Phi_t)$, $i = 1, 2, 3, 4$, i.e., $M_1 = H(\phi_{1,t})H(\phi_{2,t})H(\phi_{3,t})$, $M_2 = (1 - H(\phi_{1,t}))H(\phi_{2,t})H(\phi_{3,t})$, $M_3 = (1 - H(\phi_{2,t}))H(\phi_{3,t})$, and $M_4 = 1 - H(\phi_{3,t})$ for representing the WM, GM, CSF and background, respectively. The data fitting energy using both local intensity distribution fitting [5] and population-atlas *prior* P_i is first defined as follows,

$$E_{data}(\Phi_t) = \sum_{i=1}^{4} \int_x \Big(\int_y -K_\sigma(x - y) \log(P_i(y)p_{i,x}(\boldsymbol{I}_t(y))) M_i(\Phi_t(y)) dy \Big) dx \quad (1)$$

where x (or y) is a voxel in the image domain, K_σ is a Gaussian kernel (with scale σ) to control the size of the local region [6,7,8], $p_{i,x}(\boldsymbol{I}_t(y))$ is the probability density of $\boldsymbol{I}_t(y) = (I_{t,T1}(y), I_{t,T2}(y), I_{t,FA}(y))^T$ for the tissue class i. To take advantage of multi-modality information (T1, T2 and FA), we represent the distribution of $\boldsymbol{I}_t(y)$ as follows, with assumption that the distributions of T1, T2 and FA are independent,

$$p_{i,x}(\boldsymbol{I}_t(y)) = \prod_j p_{i,j,x}(I_{t,j}(y)) \quad (2)$$

where $p_{i,j,x}(I_{t,j}(y)) = \frac{1}{\sqrt{2\pi}\sigma_{i,j}(x)} \exp\Big(-\frac{\big(I_{t,j}(y) - \mu_{i,j}(x)\big)^2}{2\sigma_{i,j}^2(x)}\Big)$.

Note that the WM/GM contrast of the T1/T2 image is increasing/decreasing with age, implying that the weight of T1 should be higher in the adult-like stage and the weight of T2 should be higher in the infantile stage. In the isointense stage, both the contrasts of T1 and T2 images are quite low. However, the FA image shows a good contrast between WM and GM. Therefore, we propose using adaptive weights $\omega_{t,j}$ for T1, T2 and FA images in different time points, as shown in Fig. 2. Based on Eq. (2) and the adaptive weights $\omega_{t,j}$, we can further derive the data fitting term from Eq. (1) as follows,

$$E_{data}(\Phi_t) = \sum_{i=1}^{4} \int_x \Big(\int_y -K_\sigma(x-y)\big(\log P_i(y) + \sum_j \omega_{t,j} \log p_{i,j,x}(I_{t,j}(y)) \big) M_i(\Phi_t(y)) dy \Big) dx \quad (3)$$

---

[1] In this paper, the level set function takes negative values outside of the zero-level-set and positive values inside of the zero-level-set.

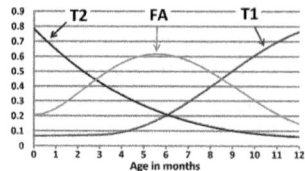

Fig. 2. The weight parameters $\omega_{t,j}$ for the T1, T2 and FA at different time points

2.2 Cortical Thickness Constraint Term

As pointed out in [9], the thickness of the cortical layer is quite consistent and can be used as a constraint to guide surface evolution. To utilize the cortical structural information, we design a coupled surface model to constrain the distance of zeros level surfaces of $\phi_{1,t}$ and $\phi_{2,t}$ within a predefined range $[d\ D]$, where $0 < d < D$. For simplicity of notation, we let $\phi_{.,t}(l)$ denote the level sets $\phi_{.,t} = l$. As illustrated in Fig. 3(a), the zero-level-sets of $\phi_{1,t}$ and $\phi_{2,t}$, i.e., $\phi_{1,t}(0)$ and $\phi_{2,t}(0)$, indicate the interfaces of WM/GM and GM/CSF boundaries, respectively. As the WM is surrounded by the GM, $\phi_{1,t}(0)$ should be interior to $\phi_{2,t}(0)$ and should fall between the level sets of $\phi_{2,t}(d)$ and $\phi_{2,t}(D)$ for achieving the reasonable thickness measures. Based on this observation, we define a new distance constraint term for $\phi_{1,t}$,

$$E_{dist}(\phi_{1,t}) = \left[1 - (H(\phi_{2,t} - d) - H(\phi_{2,t} - D))\right]\left[(H(\phi_{2,t} - d) - H(\phi_{1,t}))^2 + (H(\phi_{2,t} - D) - H(\phi_{1,t}))^2\right] \quad (4)$$

In a similar way, we can define a distance constraint term for $\phi_{2,t}$,

$$E_{dist}(\phi_{2,t}) = \left[1 - (H(\phi_{1,t} + D) - H(\phi_{1,t} + d))\right]\left[(H(\phi_{1,t} + d) - H(\phi_{2,t}))^2 + (H(\phi_{1,t} + D) - H(\phi_{2,t}))^2\right] \quad (5)$$

We use Eq. (4) to demonstrate the behavior of this distance constraint term. The term $\left[1 - (H(\phi_{2,t} - d) - H(\phi_{2,t} - D))\right]$ can be seen as a weight parameter. When the distance is within the preferred range, $\left[1 - (H(\phi_{2,t} - d) - H(\phi_{2,t} - D))\right] = 0$, then the term $E_{dist}(\phi_{1,t}) = 0$, and does not affect the propagation. When the distance is out of the preferred range, $\left[1 - (H(\phi_{2,t} - d) - H(\phi_{2,t} - D))\right] = 1$, the term $\left[(H(\phi_{2,t} - d) - H(\phi_{1,t}))^2 + (H(\phi_{2,t} - D) - H(\phi_{1,t}))^2\right]$ is activated which will constrain $\phi_{1,t}(0)$ to fall between the level sets of $\phi_{2,t}(d)$ and $\phi_{2,t}(D)$.

Therefore, we can define the following energy for initial segmentation for each time-point image,

$$E(\Phi_t) = E_{data}(\Phi_t) + \alpha\left((E_{dist}(\phi_{1,t}) + E_{dist}(\phi_{2,t})\right) + \nu E_{smooth}(\Phi_t) \quad (6)$$

where $E_{smooth}(\Phi_t) = \int \left(|\nabla H(\phi_{1,t}(x))| + |\nabla H(\phi_{2,t}(x))| + |\nabla H(\phi_{3,t}(x))|\right)dx$ is the length regularization term to maintain a smooth contour/surface during evolution, α and ν are the blending parameters. The energy (6) can only deal with a single time-point image, and thus cannot benefit from the longitudinal data. In the following, we will propose a novel longitudinally guided level sets for consistent segmentation.

2.3 Longitudinally Guided Level Set Segmentation

Anatomical structures are consistent throughout the early developmental stages [4]. Therefore, we can include a longitudinal constraint term or temporal consistency term to better guide the segmentation. For each time-point t, by using 4D

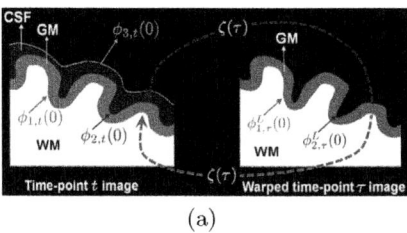 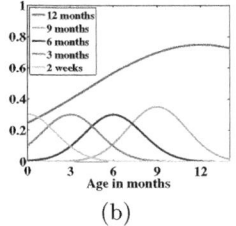

(a)   (b)

Fig. 3. (a) Longitudinal guided level-sets segmentation. (b) The weight parameters $\zeta(\tau)$ for each time-point image (the last time point is 12 months).

registration algorithm, segmentation results from other time points $\tau (\tau \neq t)$ can be registered into the space of the image at time-point t. The level set functions $\phi_{1,\tau}$ and $\phi_{2,\tau}$ can similarly be warped based on the same deformation fields. Let the warped version of $\phi_{1,\tau}$ and $\phi_{2,\tau}$ be $\phi_{1,\tau}^{L}$ and $\phi_{2,\tau}^{L}$, respectively. The distance between the zero-level-surface of $\phi_{1,t}$ (or $\phi_{2,t}$) and $\phi_{1,\tau}^{L}$ (or $\phi_{2,\tau}^{L}$) is constrained in a certain range. As illustrated in Fig. 3(a), the evolution of $\phi_{1,t}$ and $\phi_{2,t}$ is not only influenced by the information from the current image but is also adaptively constrained by longitudinal information from another time-point τ image weighted by $\zeta(\tau)$. This longitudinal constraint has a great potential to better guide tissue segmentation, and also ensure that the segmented cortical surfaces of the serial infant images are consistent with each other.

Similar to Eqs. (4) and (5), we can also constrain the distance between the zero level surfaces of $\phi_{1,t}$ (or $\phi_{2,t}$) and $\phi_{1,\tau}^{L}$ (or $\phi_{2,\tau}^{L}$). Here, we first consider $\phi_{1,t}$. Let the allowed longitudinal range of variation be $[d_1, D_1]$ with $d_1 < 0$ and $D_1 > 0$, we constrain the zero level sets $\phi_{1,t}(0)$ to fall between the level sets $\phi_{1,\tau}^{L}(d_1)$ and $\phi_{1,\tau}^{L}(D_1)$. We can define the longitudinal constraint term as,

$$E_{long}(\phi_{1,t}) = \sum_{\tau \neq t} \zeta(\tau)\left[1 - (H(\phi_{1,\tau}^{L} - d_1) - H(\phi_{1,\tau}^{L} - D_1))\right]\left[(H(\phi_{1,\tau}^{L} - d_1) - H(\phi_{1,t}))^2 \right.$$
$$\left. + (H(\phi_{1,\tau}^{L} - D_1) - H(\phi_{1,t}))^2\right] \tag{7}$$

where $\zeta(\tau)$ is the weight of each time-point, as shown in Fig. 3(b). Thus, the segmentation of each time-point image will be influenced by its neighboring time-point images. The last time-point image usually has good image contrast (see Fig. 1), therefore, its influence will be propagated further and have a greater impact on guiding the segmentation of other time-points.

Similarly, for $\phi_{2,t}$, the longitudinal constraint term can be defined as follows,

$$E_{long}(\phi_{2,t}) = \sum_{\tau \neq t} \zeta(\tau)\left[1 - (H(\phi_{2,\tau}^{L} - d_1) - H(\phi_{2,\tau}^{L} - D_1))\right]\left[(H(\phi_{2,\tau}^{L} - d_1) - H(\phi_{2,t}))^2 \right.$$
$$\left. + (H(\phi_{2,\tau}^{L} - D_1) - H(\phi_{2,t}))^2\right] \tag{8}$$

Finally, we can define the longitudinally guided level-sets energy, which combines local information from T1, T2 and FA images, cortical thickness constraint term, and longitudinal constraint term, as

$$F(\Phi_t) = E_{data}(\Phi_t) + \alpha\left(E_{dist}(\phi_{1,t}) + E_{dist}(\phi_{2,t})\right) + \beta\left(E_{long}(\phi_{1,t}) + E_{long}(\phi_{2,t})\right) + \nu E_{smooth}(\Phi_t) \tag{9}$$

where α, β and ν are the blending parameters. By calculus of variations, the energy functional $F(\Phi_t)$ (9) can be easily minimized with respect to Φ_t using the gradient descent method. The iterative procedure is presented in Algorithm. 1.

Algorithm 1. Longitudinally Guided Level Sets for Consistent Segmentation

---
Initial segmentation of each time-point using Eq. (6);
while Convergence criteria is not met **do**
    4D registration using HAMMER [10];
    Longitudinal segmentation using Eq.(9);
end while

---

3   Experimental Results

To validate our proposed method, we apply it to a group of 22 infants, each scanned at 5 time points: 2 weeks, 3, 6, 9, and 12 months (or older than 12 months). T1 images were acquired using a 3T head-only MR scanner, with 144 sagittal slices at resolution of $1{\times}1{\times}1mm^3$, TR/TE=1900/4.38ms, flip angle=7. T2 images of 64 axial slices were obtained at resolution of $1.25{\times}1.25{\times}1.95mm^3$, TR/TE=7380/119ms, flip angle=150. Preprocessing steps such as skull stripping [11] and bias correction [12] were performed. Diffusion weighted images consisting of 60 axial slices (2mm in thickness) were scanned with imaging parameters: TR/TE=7680/82ms, matrix size=128×96, 42 non-collinear diffusion gradients, diffusion weighting b=1000s/mm^2. Seven non-diffusion-weighted reference scans were also acquired. The diffusion tensor images were reconstructed and the respective FA images were computed. T2 and FA images were linearly aligned to their T1 images and were resampled with a $1{\times}1{\times}1$ mm^3 resolution before further processing. This study was approved by the ethics committee of our institute.

In our experiments, we set the allowable cortical thickness to [1, 6.5]mm, the allowable longitudinal range to [−1.5, 1.5]mm, ν=0.5, α=0.25, and β=0.5. The functions δ and H are regularized as in [13]. The level set functions are reinitialized as the signed distance functions at every iteration by using the fast marching method [14]. To measure the overlap rate between the two segmentations A and B, we employ the Dice ratio (DR), defined as $DR(A, B) = 2|A \cap B|/(|A| + |B|)$.

3.1   Single-Modality vs. Multi-modality Segmentation

To demonstrate the advantage of proposed method in terms of using T1, T2 and FA images, we first perform comparisons on the results by using T1 image only, T2 image only, which are referred to as *LongLS-T1* and *LongLS-T2*. Due to page limit, we show in Fig. 4 only the segmentation results for one subject. The original images are shown in Fig. 1. It can be clearly seen that the proposed method using T1-T2-FA yields more accurate results than the other two methods, especially the areas indicated by the red arrows and dashed curves (subcortical regions). The average DR values of the WM, GM and CSF segmentations on all 22 subjects are shown in the right of Fig. 4. It can be observed that the proposed method achieves the highest accuracy.

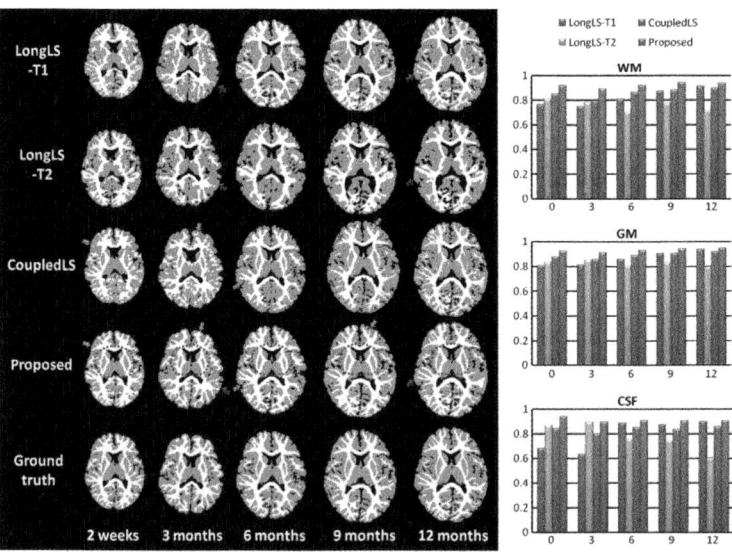

Fig. 4. *Left*: Segmentation results of *LongLS-T1*, *LongLS-T2*, the coupled level sets (CoupledLS) [5], the proposed method and ground truth. *Right*: The average Dice ratios of 22 subjects. The original images are shown in Fig. 1.

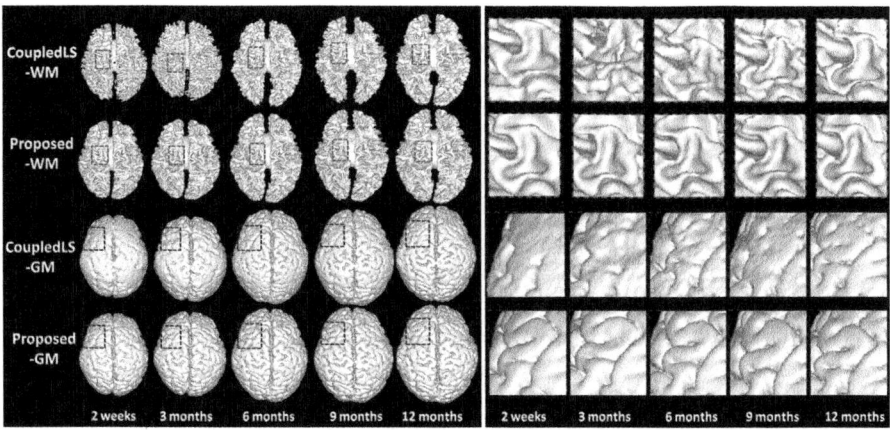

Fig. 5. Surface comparison between the coupled level sets (CoupledLS) [5] and the proposed method. The right part shows the zoomed views of the left part.

3.2   Coupled Level Sets (3D) vs. the Proposed Method (4D)

In this section, we compare the proposed method with that based on coupled level sets (CoupledLS) [5] which works only on a single time-point image and single modality. To be a fair comparison, we use multi-modality data fitting term (3) for CoupledLS. We present the segmentation results obtained by the CoupledLS in the third row of Fig. 4. It is apparent that the proposed method produce more accurate results than CoupledLS, especially at locations indicated by the green arrows. Fig. 5 shows the comparison of the 3D rendering of the WM/GM and GM/CSF surfaces. From the zoomed views (the right four columns), it can be seen that the CoupledLS cannot achieve consistent results for serial infant images, while the results of the proposed method are more consistent. The average DR values on all 22 subjects are also shown in Fig. 4, again demonstrating the advantage of the proposed method.

4   Conclusion

In this paper, we have presented a novel longitudinally guided level set method for segmentation of serial infant brain MR images. Combined information from T1, T2 and FA images are utilized by the proposed method. Longitudinal constraint is introduced to ensure consistency across time points. The proposed method has been tested on 22 subjects with promising results.

References

1. Weisenfeld, N.I., Warfield, S.K.: Automatic segmentation of newborn brain MRI. NeuroImage 47(2), 564–572 (2009)
2. Dietrich, R., et al.: MR evaluation of early myelination patterns in normal and developmentally delayed infants. AJR Am. J. Roentgenol. 150, 889–896 (1988)
3. Shi, F., et al.: Neonatal brain image segmentation in longitudinal MRI studies. NeuroImage 49(1), 391–400 (2010)
4. Armstrong, E., et al.: The ontogeny of human gyrification. Cerebral Cortex 5(1), 56–63 (1995)
5. Wang, L., et al.: Automatic segmentation of neonatal images using convex optimization and coupled level set method. In: Pan, P.J., Fan, X., Yang, Y. (eds.) MIAR 2010. LNCS, vol. 6326, pp. 1–10. Springer, Heidelberg (2010)
6. Li, C.: Active contours with local binary fitting energy. In: IMA Workshop on New Mathematics and Algorithms for 3-D Image Analysis (January 2006)
7. Li, C., et al.: Implicit active contours driven by local binary fitting energy. In: CVPR, pp. 1–7 (2007)
8. Li, C., et al.: A variational level set approach to segmentation and bias correction of images with intensity inhomogeneity. In: Metaxas, D., Axel, L., Fichtinger, G., Székely, G. (eds.) MICCAI 2008, Part II. LNCS, vol. 5242, pp. 1083–1091. Springer, Heidelberg (2008)
9. Zeng, X., et al.: Segmentation and measurement of the cortex from 3D MR images using coupled surfaces propagation. IEEE TMI 18(10), 100–111 (1999)

10. Shen, D., Davatzikos, C.: Measuring temporal morphological changes robustly in brain MR images via 4-dimensional template warping. NeuroImage 21(4), 1508–1517 (2004)
11. Shattuck, D., Leahy, R.: Automated graph-based analysis and correction of cortical volume topology. IEEE TMI 20(11), 1167–1177 (2001)
12. Sled, J., Zijdenbos, A., Evans, A.: A nonparametric method for automatic correction of intensity nonuniformity in MRI data. IEEE TMI 17(1), 87–97 (1998)
13. Chan, T., Vese, L.: Active contours without edges. IEEE TIP 10(2), 266–277 (2001)
14. Sethian, J.: Level Set Methods and Fast Marching Methods. Cambridge University Press, Cambridge (1999)

Two-Stage Multiscale Adaptive Regression Methods for Twin Neuroimaging Data

Yimei Li[1], John H. Gilmore[2], Jiaping Wang[2], Martin Styner[2], Weili Lin[2], and Hongtu Zhu[2]

[1] St. Jude Children's Research Hospital,Memphis,TN 38103
[2] University of North Carolina at Chapel Hill, Chapel Hill, NC 27599

Abstract. Twin imaging studies have been valuable for understanding the contribution of the environment and genes on brain structure and function. The conventional analyses are limited due to the same amount of smoothing throughout the whole image, the arbitrary choice of smoothing extent, and the decreased power in detecting environmental and genetic effects introduced by smoothing raw images. The goal of this article is to develop a two-stage multiscale adaptive regression method (TwinMARM) for spatial and adaptive analysis of twin neuroimaging and behavioral data. The first stage is to establish the relationship between twin imaging data and a set of covariates of interest, such as age and gender. The second stage is to disentangle the environmental and genetic influences on brain structure and function. Simulation studies and real data analysis show that TwinMARM significantly outperforms the conventional analyses.

1   Introduction

Twin neuroimaging studies have been a valuable source of information for evaluating the inheritance of brain structure and function by disentangling genetic factors from environment [1]. The standard voxel-wise methods for analyzing twin neuroimaging data on a two-dimensional (2D) surface (or in a three-dimensional (3D) volume) are sequentially executed in three steps. The first step is to use standard smoothing methods to spatially smooth the imaging data [2]. These smoothing methods apply the same amount of smoothing throughout the whole image. The second step involves fitting standard statistical models to imaging measures from all twin pairs at each voxel or surface location separately to generate a parametric map of test statistics (or p−values) [3]. The third step is to compute adjusted p-values in order to account for testing multiple hypotheses [4].The existing voxel-wise methods have three major limitations for analyzing twin neuroimaging data. First, as pointed out by [5] and many others, the voxel-wise method essentially treats all voxels as independent units, and thus it ignores the spatial coherence and spatially contiguous regions of activation with rather sharp edges existing in neuroimaging data. Second, as shown in [6], [7], the commonly used Gaussian kernel for smoothing imaging data usually blurs the image data near the edges of the significant regions, which can dramatically

T. Liu et al. (Eds.): MBIA 2011, LNCS 7012, pp. 102–109, 2011.
© Springer-Verlag Berlin Heidelberg 2011

increase the numbers of false positives and negatives. More seriously, smoothing raw imaging data can change the variance structure of imaging data, which is primarily associated with genetic and environmental factors [3].

The aim of this article is to develop a pipeline, called TwinMARM, for the spatial and adaptive analysis of twin neuroimaging data. TwinMARM consists of two stages of multiscale adaptive regression models (MARM). Each stage of TwinMARM constructs hierarchical nested spheres with increasing radius at all voxels, as well as adaptively generates weighted quasi-likelihood functions and finally efficiently utilize available information to estimate parameter estimates. Compared to standard voxel-wise approach, TwinMARM slightly increases the amount of computational time in computing parameter estimates and testing statistics, whereas it substantially outperforms the voxel-wise approach in increasing the accuracy of parameter estimates and the power of test statistics.

2 Methods

2.1 Structural Equation Model

Suppose we observe imaging measures and clinical variables from n_1 MZ twin pairs and $n_2 = n - n_1$ DZ twin pairs. Clinical variables may include some demographic and environmental variables. For notational simplicity, we assume that the $y_{ij}(v)$ are univariate imaging measures. Specifically, for the j-th subject in the i-th twin pair, we observe an $N_V \times 1$ vector of imaging measures, denoted by $Y_{ij} = \{y_{ij}(v) : v \in \mathcal{V}\}$ and a $k \times 1$ vector of clinical variables $x_{ij} = (x_{ij1}, \cdots, x_{ijk})^T$ for $i = 1, \cdots, n$ and $j = 1, 2$, where x_{ij1} is commonly set as 1 and $\mathcal{V}$ and v, respectively, represent a specific brain region and a voxel on $\mathcal{V}$. For notational simplicity, we only consider univariate measure and thus, N_V equals the number of points in $\mathcal{V}$.

At a specific voxel v, we consider the structural equation model

$$y_{ij}(v) = x_{ij}^T \boldsymbol{\beta}(v) + a_{ij}(v) + d_{ij}(v) + c_i(v) + e_{ij}(v), \tag{1}$$

for $j = 1, 2$ and $i = 1, \cdots, n = n_1 + n_2$, where $\boldsymbol{\beta}(v) = (\beta_1(v), \cdots, \beta_k(v))^T$ is a $k \times 1$ vector representing unknown regression coefficients, $a_{ij}(v)$, $d_{ij}(v)$, $c_i(v)$ and $e_{ij}(v)$ are, respectively, the additive genetic, dominance genetic, common environmental, and residual effects on the i-th twin pair. It is common to assume that $a_{ij}(v)$, $d_{ij}(v)$, $c_i(v)$ and $e_{ij}(v)$ are independently normally distributed with mean 0 and variance $\sigma_a(v)^2$, $\sigma_d(v)^2$, $\sigma_c(v)^2$, and $\sigma_e(v)^2$, respectively [8], [3]. Moreover, $\text{Cov}(a_{i1}(v), a_{i2}(v))$ equals $\sigma_a(v)^2$ for MZ twins and $\sigma_a(v)^2/2$ for DZ twins, while $\text{Cov}(d_{i1}(v), d_{i2}(v))$ equals $\sigma_d(v)^2$ for MZ twins and $\sigma_d(v)^2/4$ for DZ twins [9]. Due to the identifiability issue, we focus on ACE model from now on.

2.2 TwinMARM

We propose the TwinMARM for the analysis of twin imaging and behavioral data as follows. The first stage is to estimate $\boldsymbol{\beta} = \{\boldsymbol{\beta}(v) : v \in \mathcal{V}\}$, while the second stage is to estimate $\boldsymbol{\eta} = \{\boldsymbol{\eta}(v) = (\sigma_a(v)^2, \sigma_c(v)^2, \sigma_e(v)^2)^T : v \in \mathcal{V}\}$. In each stage, we reformulate the problem of estimating $\boldsymbol{\beta}$ (or $\boldsymbol{\eta}$) as a regression model and then apply the MARM, which is a generalization of the propogation-seperation (PS) procedure in multiple subjects [10], [11]. The key ideas of MARM (or PS) are to construct hierarchical nested spheres with increasing radius at all voxels, to adaptively construct weighted quasi-likelihood functions to estimate parameter estimates and thus to increase the power of test statistics in detecting subtle changes of brain structure and function.

TwinMARM: Stage I We consider a bivariate regression model given by

$$Y_i(v) = \begin{pmatrix} y_{i1}(v) \\ y_{i2}(v) \end{pmatrix} = \mathbf{x}_i^T \boldsymbol{\beta}(v) + \mathbf{f}_i(v) = \begin{pmatrix} \mathbf{x}_{i1}^T \\ \mathbf{x}_{i2}^T \end{pmatrix} \boldsymbol{\beta}(v) + \begin{pmatrix} f_{i1}(v) \\ f_{i2}(v) \end{pmatrix}, \qquad (2)$$

where $\mathbf{x}_i = [\mathbf{x}_{i1} \; \mathbf{x}_{i2}]$ and $\mathbf{f}_i(v) = (f_{i1}(v), f_{i2}(v))^T$, in which $f_{ij}(v) = a_{ij}(v) + c_i(v) + e_{ij}(v)$ for ACE model. Although $\mathbf{f}_i(v)$ has different covariance structures for MZ and DZ, respectively, we assume that $\mathbf{f}_i(v)$ has mean zero and covariance $\Sigma_f(v)$ for all i to avoid estimating variance components $(\sigma_a(v)^2, \sigma_c(v)^2, \sigma_e(v)^2)$ in Stage I, which leads a simple procedure for making inference on β. We will appropriately account for the misspecification of covariance of $\mathbf{f}_i(v)$ in our statistical inference on $\boldsymbol{\beta}(v)$.

Since all components of $\boldsymbol{\beta}(v)$ are the parameters of interest and $\Sigma_f(v)$ can be regarded as nuisance parameters, we first estimate $\Sigma_f(v)$ across all voxels and then fix them at their estimated values. We calculate the maximum pseudo-likelihood estimate based on the following pseudo-likelihood of $Y_i(v)$ given $\mathbf{x}_i$ given by

$$-0.5 \log |\Sigma_f(v)| - 0.5\{Y_i(v) - \mathbf{x}_i^T \boldsymbol{\beta}(v)\}^T \Sigma_f(v)^{-1} \{Y_i(v) - \mathbf{x}_i^T \boldsymbol{\beta}(v)\}. \qquad (3)$$

From now on, $\Sigma_f(v)$ will be fixed at $\hat{\Sigma}_f(v)$ across all voxels v.

To estimate $\boldsymbol{\beta}(v)$ at voxel v, we construct a weighted quasi-likelihood function by utilizing all imaging data in a sphere with radius h at voxel v, denoted by $B(v, h)$. Let $\omega(v, v'; h) \in [0, 1]$ be a weight function of two voxels and a radius h, which characterizes the similarity between the data in voxels v and v' such that $\omega(v, v; h) = 1$ for all $h > 0$. If $\omega(v, v'; h) \approx 1$, it represents that the data in voxels v and v' are very close to each other, whereas $\omega(v, v'; h) \approx 0$ indicates that the data in voxel v' do not contain too much information on $\boldsymbol{\beta}(v)$. The adaptive weights $\omega(v, v'; h)$ play an important role in preventing oversmoothing the estimates of $\boldsymbol{\beta}(v)$ as well as preserving the edges of significant regions. We utilize all the data $\{Y_i(v') : v' \in B(v, h)\}$ to construct the weighted log-likelihood function at voxel v at scale h, denoted by $\ell_{obs}(\boldsymbol{\beta}(v); h)$ as follows:

$$-0.5 \sum_{i=1}^{n} \sum_{v' \in B(v,h)} \omega(v, v'; h) \{Y_i(v) - \mathbf{x}_i^T \boldsymbol{\beta}(v)\}^T \hat{\Sigma}_f(v')^{-1} \{Y_i(v) - \mathbf{x}_i^T \boldsymbol{\beta}(v)\}. \quad (4)$$

By maximizing $\ell_{obs}(\boldsymbol{\beta}(v); h)$, we obtain the maximum pseudo-likelihood estimate of $\boldsymbol{\beta}(v)$, denoted by $\hat{\boldsymbol{\beta}}(v; h)$, and thus obtain its covariance matrix $\Sigma_n(\hat{\boldsymbol{\beta}}(v; h))$.

We can further construct test statistic to test scientific questions about $\beta(v)$. These questions usually can be formulated as $H_{0,\mu} : R\beta = \mathbf{b}_0$ versus $H_{1,\mu} : R\beta \neq \mathbf{b}_0$, where R is an $r \times q$ matrix and b_0 is an $r \times 1$ vector. We test the null hypothesis $H_{0,\mu} : R\beta(v) = 0$ using the Wald test statistic $W_\mu(v;h) = [R\hat{\beta}(v;h) - \mathbf{b}_0]^T [R\Sigma_n(\hat{\beta}(v;h))R^T]^{-1}[R\hat{\beta}(v;h) - \mathbf{b}_0]$.

Adaptive Estimation and Testing Procedure. The key idea of AET is to build a sequence of nested spheres with increasing radii $h_0 = 0 < h_1 < \cdots < h_S = r_0$ at each voxel $v \in \mathcal{V}$. As $h = h_1$, we extract features from the imaging data as well as $\{\hat{\beta}(v;h_0) : v \in \mathcal{V}\}$ and compute weights $\omega(v,v';h_1)$ at scale h_1 for all $v, v' \in \mathcal{V}$. Then, we adaptively determine $\omega(v,v';h_s)$ and update $\hat{\beta}(v;h_s)$ and $W_\mu(v,h_s)$ from h_1 to $h_S = r_0$. A path diagram is given below:

$$\{\hat{\beta}(v) : v \in \mathcal{V}\} \Rightarrow \quad \omega(v,v';h_1) \qquad \cdots \qquad \omega(v,v';h_S = r_0)$$
$$\Downarrow \qquad \nearrow \cdots \nearrow \qquad \qquad \Downarrow$$
$$\{\hat{\beta}(v;h_1) : v \in \mathcal{V}\} \quad \cdots \quad \{(\hat{\beta}(v;h_S), W_\mu(v;h_S)) : v \in \mathcal{V}\}.$$

TwinMARM: Stage II Given $\{\hat{\beta}(v;S) : v \in \mathcal{V}\}$ obtained from Stage I, we compute residuals $\hat{r}_{ij}(v) = y_{ij}(v) - \mathbf{x}_i^T \hat{\beta}(v;S)$ for all i,j across all $v \in \mathcal{V}$. Then, we consider a trivariate regression model given by

$$\mathbf{r}_i(v) = \begin{pmatrix} \hat{r}_{i1}(v)^2 \\ \hat{r}_{i2}(v)^2 \\ \hat{r}_{i1}(v)\hat{r}_{i2}(v) \end{pmatrix} = \mathbf{z}_i^T \boldsymbol{\eta}(v) + \mathbf{e}_i(v) = \begin{pmatrix} \mathbf{z}_{i1}^T \\ \mathbf{z}_{i2}^T \\ \mathbf{z}_{i3}^T \end{pmatrix} \boldsymbol{\eta}(v) + \begin{pmatrix} e_{i1}(v) \\ e_{i2}(v) \\ e_{i3}(v) \end{pmatrix}, \quad (5)$$

where $\mathbf{e}_i(v) = (e_{i1}(v), e_{i2}(v), e_{i3}(v))^T$ and $\mathbf{z}_i = [\mathbf{z}_{i1}\ \mathbf{z}_{i2}\ \mathbf{z}_{i3}]$, in which $\mathbf{z}_{i1} = \mathbf{z}_{i2} = (1,1,1)^T$ and $\mathbf{z}_{i3}$ equals $(0.5,1,0)$ for DZ and $(1,1,0)$ for MZ. Moreover, $\mathbf{e}_i(v)$ is assumed to have mean zero and covariance $\Sigma_e(v)$ for all i. Since models (2) and (5) are similar in nature, we omit the detail for the sake of simplicity. There is a minor difference between models (2) and (5). In model (5), all regression coefficients in $\boldsymbol{\eta}(v)$ are constrained to be non-negative. We employ a hinge algorithm for cone projection [12]. See for example [13] and among many others, we can form a Wald test statistic $W_A(v;h)$ similar to those in Stage I to test genetic and environmental influence on brain structure and function. Moreover, the AET procedure in Stage I can be applied here to spatially and adaptively estimate $\boldsymbol{\eta}(v)$ and carry out statistical inference on $\boldsymbol{\eta}(v)$.

3   Results

Simulation Studies. We simulated MRI measures from n pairs of siblings according to ACE model, in which $\beta(v) = (\beta_1(v), \beta_2(v), \beta_3(v))^T$ and $x_{ij} = (x_{1ij}, x_{2ij}, x_{3ij})^T$. Each family contained only two siblings. Among the n pairs of twins, 60% are identical twins. We set $x_{1ij} \equiv 1$, generated x_{2ij} independently from a Bernoulli distribution, with probability of success 0.5, and generated x_{3ij} independently from the Gaussian distribution with zero mean and unit variance.

The x_{2ij} and x_{3ij} were chosen to represent gender identity and scaled age respectively. We set $(\beta_2(v), \beta_3(v), \sigma_d(v)^2, \sigma_e(v)^2)^T = (1, 1, 1, 1)^T$ across all voxels v. For $(\beta_1(v), \sigma_a(v)^2)$, we divided the 64×64 phantom image into five different regions of interest (ROIs) with different shapes and then varied $(\beta_1(v), \sigma_a(v)^2)$ as $(0, 0), (0.3, 0.5), (0.6, 1), (0.9, 1.5)$ and $(1.2, 2.0)$ across these five ROIs. The true $(\beta_1(v), \sigma_a(v)^2)$ was displayed for all ROIs with black, blue, red, yellow, and white colors representing $(\beta_1(v), \sigma_a(v)^2) = (0, 0), (0.3, 0.5), (0.6, 1), (0.9, 1.5)$ and $(1.2, 2.0)$ (Fig. 2 (A) and (E)). We generated $\mathbf{e}_i(v) = (e_{i1}(v), e_{i2}(v))^T$, $\mathbf{a}_i(v) = (a_{i1}(v), a_{i2}(v))^T$, and $c_i(v)$ independently from multivariate Gaussian generators with zero means and covariance matrices as specified in Section 2.1. We set $n = 100$ and 400.

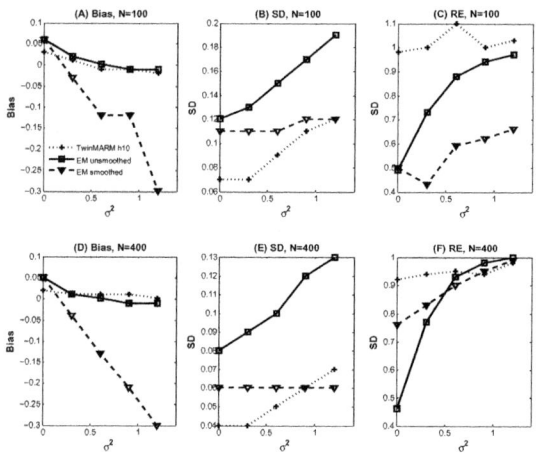

Fig. 1. Results from a simulation study of comparing EM and TwinMARM at 2 different sample sizes ($n = 100, 400$). The first row contains the results for $\sigma_a(v)^2$ as $n = 100$: Panel (A) is the bias curve of $\sigma_a(v)^2 = 0$, 0.5, 1.0, 1.5 and 2.0, respectively. Panel (B) is the SD curve of $\hat{\sigma}_a(v; h_{10})^2$ obtained from a simulated dataset by using TwinMARM, EM, and EM with smoothed data. Panel (C) is the ratio of RMS over SD. The second row contains panels (D), (E), and (F) as $n = 400$, which are the corresponding results of panels of panels (A), (B), and (C) respectively.

We fitted the structural equation model $y_{ij}(v) = \mathbf{x}_{ij}^T \beta(v) + a_{ij}(v) + c_i(v) + e_{ij}(v)$, in which the correlation pattern of $a_{ij}(v)$, $c_i(v)$ and $e_{ij}(v)$ was specified according to Secion 2.1. We calculated the maximum likelihood estimates (MLEs) of $(\beta(v), \sigma_a(v)^2, \sigma_e(v)^2, \sigma_c(v)^2)^T$ at each pixel by using the expectation-maximization (EM) algorithm [14]. Then, we applied the TwinMARM procedure to calculate adaptive parameter estimates across all pixels at 11 different scales. We also smoothed the subjects' images by using an isotropic Gaussian kernel with FWHM 3 pixels and then applied the EM algorithm to the smoothed data. Furthermore, for $(\beta_1(v), \sigma_a(v)^2)$, we calculated the bias, the empirical standard error RMS, the mean of the standard error estimates SD, and the ratio of RMS

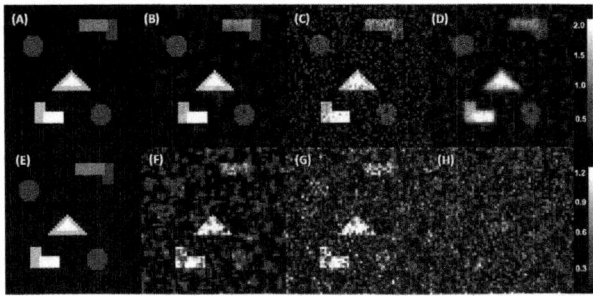

Fig. 2. Simulation study. First row: Panel (A) is the ground truth image of five ROIs with black, blue, red, yellow, and white color representing $\beta_1(v)$=0, 0.3, 0.6, 0.9, and 1.2, respectively. Panel (B) is a selected slice of $\hat{\beta}_2(d, h_{10})$ obtained by TwinMARM method from a simulated dataset. Panel (C) is a selected slice of $\hat{\beta}_2(v)$ by voxel-wise method obtained from the same dataset used in panel (B). Panel (D) is a selected slice of $\hat{\beta}_2(v)$ by the voxel-wise method, after we directly smoothed the same simulated dataset as the one used in panel (B). Second row: Panel (E) is the ground truth image of five ROIs with black, blue, red, yellow, and white color representing $\sigma_a(v)^2$=0, 0.5, 1.0, 1.5, and 2.0, respectively. Panel (F) is a selected slice of $\hat{\sigma}_a(d, h_{10})^2$ obtained by TwinMARM method from a simulated dataset. Panel (G) is a selected slice of $\hat{\sigma}_a^2(v)$ by voxel-wise method obtained from the same dataset as (F). Panel (H) is a selected slice of $\hat{\sigma}_a(v)^2$ by the voxel-wise method, after we smoothed the same simulated data set as (F).

over SD, abbreviated as RE at each pixel of all five ROIs based on the results obtained from the 1000 simulated data sets. For simplicity, we present some selected results for $\hat{\beta}_1(v; h)$ and $\hat{\sigma}_a^2(v; h)$ and their corresponding MLEs obtained from the EM algorithm with smoothed and unsmoothed data. We considered $\hat{\sigma}_a(v; h)^2$ as an example. The biases of $\hat{\sigma}_a(v; h)^2$ are almost the same for Twin-MARM at h_{10} and EM with unsmoothed data, while the bias from EM with smoothed data is greatly increased (Fig. 1 (A) and (D)). Inspecting the results from the EM algorithm reveals that SD is consistently larger than that obtained from TwinMARM at h_{10} (Fig. 1 (B) and (E)). The ratio of RMS over SD, abbreviated as RE is displayed in (Fig. 1 (C) and (F)). The RE is closed to 1 for TwinMARM for both sample size. TwinMARM outperforms EM in terms of smaller RMS (Fig. 2 (F) and (G)) . Similarly, TwinMARM outperforms EM in terms of smaller RMS for estimating $\beta_1(v)$ (Fig. 2 (B) and (C)).

Real Data. We considered the early postnatal brain development project and a total of 49 paired twins (36 males and 62 females) were selected. All 49 pairs were scanned as neonates within a few weeks after birth at term. We used a 3T Allegra head-only MR system (Siemens) to acquire all the images. We used a single shot EPI DTI sequence (TR/TE=5400/73 msec) with eddy current compensation to acquire the DTI images. The acquisition sequence consists of five repetitions of six gradient scans (b = 1000 s/mm^2) at non-collinear directions and a single reference scan (in total 5x7 = 35 images). The voxel resolution was isotropic 2 mm, and the in-plane field of view was set at 256 mm in both directions. We then estimated diffusion tensor images and employed a nonlinear fluid deformation based high- dimensional, unbiased atlas computation method to process all 98 DTI datasets.

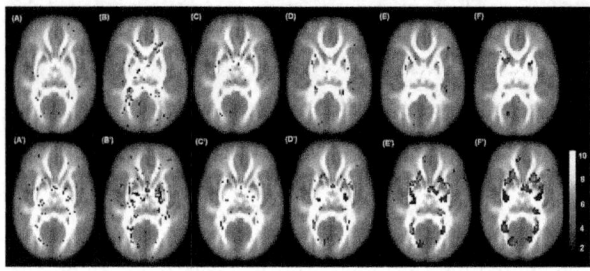

Fig. 3. Results from the 49 twin pairs in a neonatal project on brain development on the selected 27th and 30th slices. Panels (A)-(F) : the $-\log_{10}(p)$ values for testing genetic effects by using TwinMARM at the 1st and 10th iterations and EM with FWHM equal to 0mm, 3mm, 6mm, 9mm for the 27th slice ; Panels (A')-(F') : the corresponding $-\log_{10}(p)$ values for testing environmental effects for the 30th slice.

We considered a linear model $y_{ij}(v) = \beta_1(v) + \beta_2(v)G_{ij} + \beta_3(v)Z_{ij} + a_{ij}(v) + c_i(v) + \epsilon_{ij}(v)$ for $i = 1, \cdots, 49$ and $j = 1, 2$ at each voxel of the template, where G_{ij} and Z_{ij}, respectively, represent the dummy variables for gender (male=1 and female=0) and zygote (MZ=1 and DZ=0), and $a_{ij}(v)$, $c_i(v)$ and $e_{ij}(v)$ are, respectively, the additive genetic, common environmental, and residual effects on the i-th twin pair. We focused on the major white matter regions. We calculated the MLE of parameters by using the EM algorithm with unsmoothed or smoothed data and also applied our TwinMARM method with $c_h = 1.15$ and $S = 10$ to carry out statistical analysis. We tested $H_0 : \sigma_a(v)^2 = 0$ for additive genetic effect across all voxels v in the white matter regions. To correct for multiple comparisons, we used the raw p-value smaller than 0.05 along with a 20 voxel extent threshold. We found significant regions in the inferior frontal gyrus, triangular part and mid cingulate cortex regions. We identified more voxels by using TwinMARM compared to EM. We also tested $H_0 : \sigma_c(v)^2 = 0$ for common environmental effect across all voxels v. Several interesting regions identified included the the right precentral gyrus, inferior frontal gyrus, triangular part, supplementary motor area, insula, hippocampus, right fusiform, and thalamus. Fig. 3 show some selected slices of $-\log_{10}(p)$ map for environmental effect obtained from the 10th iteration of TwinMARM. The results clearly show that TwinMARM has significantly improved sensitivity and reliability as areas of significance in the TwinMARM results appear larger and smoother compared to the voxel-wise analysis approach, which is close to the result obtained from the first iteration of TwinMARM. The results from EM with smoothed data from FWHM=6mm and 9mm may possibly include some false positive results (Fig. 3).

Acknowledgements. This work was supported in part by NIH grants RR025747-01, P01CA142538-01, MH086633, and AG033387 to Dr. Zhu, NIH grants MH064065, HD053000, and MH070890 to Dr. Gilmore, NIH grants R01NS055754 and R01EB5-34816 to Dr. Lin, Lilly Research Laboratories, the UNC NDRC HD 03110, Eli Lilly grant F1D-MC-X252, and NIH Roadmap Grant U54 EB005149-01, NAMIC to Dr. Styner.

References

1. Thompson, P.M., Cannon, T.D., Narr, K.L., van Erp, T., Poutanen, V., Huttunen, M., Lonnqvist, J., Standertskjold-Nordenstam, C.G., Kaprio, J., Khaledy, M., Dail, R., Zoumalan, C.I., Toga, A.: Genetic inuences on brain structure. Nature Neuroscience 4, 1253–1358 (2001)
2. Yoon, U., Fahim, C., Perusse, D., Evans, A.C.: Lateralized genetic and environmental inuences on human brain morphology of 8-year-old twins. NeuroImage 53, 1117–1125 (2010)
3. Neale, M.C., Heath, A.C., Hewitt, J.K., Eaves, L.J., Fulker, D.W.: Fitting genetic models with lisrel: Hypothesis testing. Behavior Genetics 19, 37–49 (1989)
4. Nichols, T., Hayasaka, S.: Controlling the familywise error rate in functional neuroimaging: a comparative review. Stat. Methods Med. Res. 12, 419–426 (2003)
5. Worsley, K.J., Taylor, J.E., Tomaiuolo, F., Lerch, J.: Unified univariate and multivariate random field theory. NeuroImage 23, 189–195 (2004)
6. Polzehl, J., Spokoiny, V.G.: Adaptive weights smoothing with applications to image restoration. J. R. Statist. Soc. B 62, 335–354 (2000)
7. Qiu, P.: Image Processing and Jump Regression Analysis. John Wiley & Sons, New York (2005)
8. Feng, R., Zhou, G., Zhang, M., Zhang, H.: Analysis of twin data using sas. Biometrics 65, 584–589 (2009)
9. Falconer, D.S., Mackay, T.F.C.: Introduction to Quantitative Genetics. Longman, Harlow (1996)
10. Tabelow, K., Polzehl, J., Voss, H.U., Spokoiny, V.: Analyzing fmri experiments with structural adaptive smoothing procedures. NeuroImage 33, 55–62 (2006)
11. Tabelow, K., Polzehl, J., Ulug, A.M., Dyke, J.P., Watts, R., Heier, L.A., Voss, H.U.: Accurate localization of brain activity in presurgical fmri by structure adaptive smoothing. IEEE Trans. Med. Imaging 27, 531–537 (2008)
12. Meyer, M.C.: An algorithm for quadratic programming with applications in statistics (2009)
13. Thompson, P.M., Cannon, T.D., Toga, A.W.: Mapping genetic inuences on human brain structure. Ann. Med. 24, 523–536 (2002)
14. Dempster, A.P., Laird, N.M., Rubin, D.B.: Maximum likelihood from incomplete data via the em algorithm. Journal of the Royal Statistical Society, Series B 39, 1–38 (1977)

Segmentation of Medical Images of Different Modalities Using Distance Weighted C-V Model

Xiaozheng Liu[1,4], Wei Liu[1], Yan Xu[1], Yongdi Zhou[2], Junming Zhu[3], Bradley S. Peterson[4], and Dongrong Xu[4,*]

[1] Key Laboratory of Brain Functional Genomics, Ministry of Education, China & Shanghai Key Laboratory of Brain Functional Genomics, East China Normal University, Shanghai Key Laboratory of Magnetic Resonance, East China Normal University, Shanghai 20062, China
[2] Department of Neurosurgery, Johns Hopkins University, Baltimore, MD 21287, USA
[3] Department of Neurosurgery, The Second Affiliated Hospital of Zhejiang University, Hangzhou 310009, China
[4] MRI Unit, Columbia University Dept of Psychiatry, & New York State Psychiatric Institute, NYSPI Unit 74, 1051 Riverside Drive, New York, NY 10032, USA
dx2103@columbia.edu

Abstract. Region-based active contour model (ACM) has been extensively used in medical image segmentation and Chan & Vese's (C-V) model is one of the most popular ACM methods. We propose to incorporate into the C-V model a weighting function to take into consideration the fact that different locations in an image with differing distances from the active contour have differing importance in generating the segmentation result, thereby making it a weighted C-V (WC-V) model. The theoretical properties of the model and our experiments both demonstrate that the proposed WC-V model can significantly reduce the computational cost while improve the accuracy of segmentation over the results using the C-V model.

1 Introduction

Segmentation is an important preprocessing step in many image analysis tasks ranging from spatial normalization to robot navigation. The result of image segmentation is usually the basis of those advanced further studies that employ imaging data, such as diagnosis, localization of pathology, surgical and treatment planning, and therapy evaluation. Because medical images are vulnerable to a number of factors, including image noise, occluded structures, imaging inhomogeneity and partial volume effects, accurate segmentation of medical images remains a challenging topic in practice.

A great number of techniques have been developed and documented for medical image segmentation [3,4]. Active contour model (ACM) [1,2,5-13] using level set [7] is one of the most successful methods. Mathematically, each ACM corresponds to a variational function binding with certain constraints that associate to the nature of the target object in the image to be segmented. Minimizing this function in terms of the energy of the constraints, ACM generates a curve in a 2D image plane which evolves to

---

* Corresponding author.

T. Liu et al. (Eds.): MBIA 2011, LNCS 7012, pp. 110–117, 2011.
© Springer-Verlag Berlin Heidelberg 2011

extract the object under detection. In general, ACM methods in the literatures can be classified into two major classes: edge-based models [5,6] and region-based models [2,8-11].

The edge-based models mainly use image gradient as a powerful constraint to stop the evolving curve on the boundaries of the target objects. Usually, a stopping function based on the image gradient is needed to move the contours towards the desired boundaries. However, the image gradient is unable to move a contour far from the actual boundary in a homogeneous area where the gradient is zero. In addition, noise and false boundaries may create numerous local minima that could easily trap the moving contour [10]. In contrast, region-based models use region-related information to construct constraints, thus may overcome the drawbacks of edge-based models in this aspect. These methods do not use the image gradient to drive the contour curve, therefore, they can work in the image where objects only show weak or even invisible boundaries. Moreover, the segmentation contour can be initialized anywhere in the image, without worrying it being trapped in areas of zero-gradient. The region-based C-V models are therefore generally superior to the edge-based models for image segmentation. One of the most popular region-based models is the C-V model [2], which is based on the Mumford-Shan segmentation techniques [2] and has been successfully used in binary phase segmentation under an assumption that each image region is statistically homogeneous. Certainly, the C-V model does not work well for images with significantly inhomogeneous intensities. Moreover, the computational cost of the C-V model is exceptionally high, usually unacceptable for real-time applications of image segmentation.

To improve the accuracy of segmentation using C-V model, local region C-V model utilizing the local image information (for example, information in a small neighborhood immediately next to the active contour instead of all the voxels in the whole region either inside or outside of the contour) can achieve relatively more accurate results in segmenting images with inhomogeneous intensity than does the conventional C-V model [8-11]. Studies using such a local region model actually demonstrated that the neighborhood of the active contour has a large effect on segmentation accuracy. To boost the efficiency of the C-V model, several methods proposed to replace the continuous variational formulation of the level set using discrete steps, assigning different values to coordinate points according to whose locations are closer to or farther away from the active contour [12,12]. However, the models of these proposed revisions were too complex to be incorporated directly into the equations of level set. Nevertheless, these work demonstrated that points at different locations should have different effects on the segmentation procedure depending on their relative distances from the active contour. This observation therefore led us to the development of a continuous weighting function to be embedded into the C-V model for improved segmentation accuracy and efficiency. We name this model as a weighted C-V (WC-V) model. Our method is hopefully to move the active contour aggressively toward the true boundary so that the segmentation procedure will evolve much faster and more accurate than does the conventional C-V models.

2   The C-V Model

An ACM based on the Mumford Shah model was proposed [2] for a special case that the image is piecewise constant (i.e., intensities are locally constant in connected regions). Let I: $\Omega \rightarrow R$ be an input image (Ω the image domain and R the set of real values) and C be a closed curve, the energy functional is defined as:

$$E^{CV}(C,c_1,c_2) = \mu \cdot length(C) + v \cdot area(inside(C))$$
$$+ \lambda_1 \int_{inside(C)} |I - c_1|^2 \, dx + \lambda_2 \int_{outside(C)} |I - c_2|^2 \, dx, \quad x \in \Omega \tag{1}$$

where $\mu \geq 0, v \geq 0, \lambda_1, \lambda_2 > 0$ are fixed parameters. The μ and v are zero or positive values to control the effect of the first two terms in minimizing the function. c_1 and c_2 are two updating values that approximate the average image intensities inside and outside the contour C, respectively.

The above energy functional can be solved under the framework of level set [7], in which the contour C is presented by the zero level set of a real-valued Lipschitz function ϕ, such that $C = \{x \in \Omega \mid \phi(x) = 0\}$. By minimizing the above energy functional through the gradient descent method with respect to the constants c_1 and c_2, the energy function $E^{cv}(C,c_1,c_2)$ can be reformulated as the following variational formulation:

$$c_1(\phi) = \frac{\int_\Omega IH(\phi)d\Omega}{\int_\Omega H(\phi)d\Omega}, \quad c_2(\phi) = \frac{\int_\Omega I(1-H(\phi))d\Omega}{\int_\Omega (1-H(\phi))d\Omega} \tag{2}$$

$$\frac{\partial \phi}{\partial t} = \delta(\phi)[\mu div(\frac{\nabla \phi}{|\nabla \phi|}) - v - \lambda_1(I-c_1)^2 + \lambda_2(I-c_2)^2] \tag{3}$$

where $H(\phi)$ and $\delta(\phi)$ are the regularized approximation of Heaviside function and Dirac delta function respectively [2].

3   Our Method

3.1   WC-V Model

Because the points near the active contour should be more important than the points away from the active contour for evolving the contour, we add a weighting term to the C-V model. This term should be able to assign weights to the points according to their relative locations to the active contour. Our weighting function is thus defined as:

$$w(x,\phi) = \exp(-\alpha \cdot d(x,\phi(x) = 0)) \tag{4}$$

where $d(x,\phi(x) = 0)$ is the distance between point x and the active contour, and α is the parameters for adjustment of the weighting amplitude.

Actually, the level set function ϕ includes the distance information between point x [14] and active contour, so we represent $d(x,\phi(x) = 0)$ as absolute value of ϕ in Eq. (4). Then the weighting function becomes $w(x,\phi) = \exp(-\alpha \cdot abs(\phi))$.

The WC-V model is therefore defined as:

$$E^{WCV}(C,c_1,c_2) = \mu \cdot length(C) + v \cdot area(inside(C))$$
$$+\lambda_1 \int_{inside(C)} w(x,\phi)|I(x)-c_1|^2 \, dx + \lambda_2 \int_{outside(C)} w(x,\phi)|I(x)-c_2|^2 \, dx, \quad x \in \Omega \qquad (5)$$

where $\mu \geq 0, v \geq 0, \lambda_1, \lambda_2 > 0$ are fixed parameters, I: $\Omega \rightarrow R$ is an input image.

Similar to the C-V model [2], minimizing the above energy functional with respect to ϕ leads to the steepest descent flow as follows:

$$c_1(\phi) = \frac{\int_\Omega w(x)I(x)H(\phi)d\Omega}{\int_\Omega w(x)H(\phi)d\Omega}, \quad c_2(\phi) = \frac{\int_\Omega w(x)I(x)(1-H(\phi))d\Omega}{\int_\Omega w(x)(1-H(\phi))d\Omega} \qquad (6)$$

$$\frac{\partial \phi}{\partial t} = \delta(\phi)[\mu \, div(\frac{\nabla \phi}{|\nabla \phi|}) - v - w(x,\phi)\lambda_1(I(x)-c_1)^2 + w(x,\phi)\lambda_2(I(x)-c_2)^2$$
$$+\alpha w(x,\phi)H(\phi)\lambda_1(I(x)-c_1)^2 - \alpha w(x,\phi)(1-H(\phi))\lambda_2(I(x)-c_2)^2] \qquad (7)$$

Compared with the C-V model, c_1 and c_2 in our WC-V model become the weighted mean intensities inside and outside the contour C, respectively.

3.2   Implementation

All the partial derivatives in Eq. (7) can be discretized simply using central finite differences. The temporal derivative is discretized as a forward difference, an iterative scheme is therefore obtained by discretizing Eq. (7). We initialize the level set function ϕ as a binary function that denotes points inside the initial contour to be 1 and outside 0.

In the iterative process, we reinitialize the evolved level values defined by ϕ every few iterations as required by the algorithm using a fast marching scheme [14] to guarantee that ϕ approximates to a signed distance function that satisfies the Eikonal Equation $|\nabla \phi|=1$ [7].

3.3   Experiment Design

Our algorithm was implemented in Matlab 2008b on a 2.8-GHz intel Pentium IV personal computer. We applied our method to medical images using the same set of parameters ($\lambda_1 = \lambda_2 = 1$, $v = 0$, $\mu = 0.02$) and the Courant-Friedrichs-Levy condition [14] as our time-step. In our experiments, we set $\alpha = 0.1$.

We compared the performance of three models: the conventional C-V model, a local region active contour model (LAC) [9] and WC-V model. For LCV model, the size of the neighborhood needed to be adjusted in the experiments depending on the nature of the images.

In the first experiment, we would like to compare the performance of three methods using data from 3 different imaging modalities (Fig.1) : a slice of a cardiac magnetic resonance (MR) image containing the left ventricles of a human heart; an ultrasound image of the same organ but from a different sectional view and a Computer Tomography (CT) image of human lungs. We aimed to use the algorithms to segment the ventricles and the lungs in these images.

In the second experiment, we wanted to examine and compare the performance of the 3 methods using MR images with different levels of noise and intensity non-uniformities. We used midsaggital images with differing levels of noise and tested on them using the algorithms to segment the corpus callosum (CC), because the CC is a well-known and important structure, serving as the major connectivity pathway between the two cerebral hemispheres, and most of the communications between regions in the two halves of the brain are carried over the CC [15].We downloaded 10 datasets of brain images from the McGill Brain Web [16], each containing three brain images of the same person differing only the noise level (0%,5%,9%) and intensity non-uniformity (0%,20%,40%) (Fig. 2). Two experienced human experts on brain anatomy manually segmented the brain and their average formed a CC template to be used as the standard reference. The Root Square Error $(RSE) = \sqrt{\sum |M(x) - M_o(x)|^2}$ between this reference and the results generated by the 3 methods was used for quantitative comparison of the segmentation performance, in which $M(x)$ is the result generated by different approaches, $M_0(x)$ the manual reference. The smaller the RSE was, the better agreement between the reference and the generated result.

We conducted visual inspection and comparisons for both experiments. We also checked the computational costs by comparing the number of iterations and CPU time needed for convergence of the active contour.

4   Experiment Results

The first experiment demonstrated that our WC-V method generated more accurate results than did other models on all the 3 types of medical images (Fig. 1). Compared with the results by the other two models, the boundaries generated by the WC-V model obviously agreed better to the truth that human anatomists can identify, particularly in regions with rich details (Fig.1); whereas the C-V model could only roughly separate the ventricles in the cardiac images and the lungs in the CT image, missing lots delicate details. Moreover, the LCV model was sensitive to disturbances arising from small structures that were not riding on tissue boundary but in locations with rich local details (greed arrow in Fig 1).

The second experiment demonstrated that the WC-V model worked efficiently and equally well at differing levels of noise and intensity non-uniformity (Table 2). Both the WC-V model and LCV models obtained results that were roughly correct (Fig 2)⁐ however, the boundary generated by LCV model was relatively noisy (Fig 2), and the RSE of using the WC-V model is smaller (Table 2). In contrast, the results generated using the C-V model varied significantly across different noise and non-uniformity levels. It seems that the C-V model is very unstable because the results varied significantly (Fig. 2).

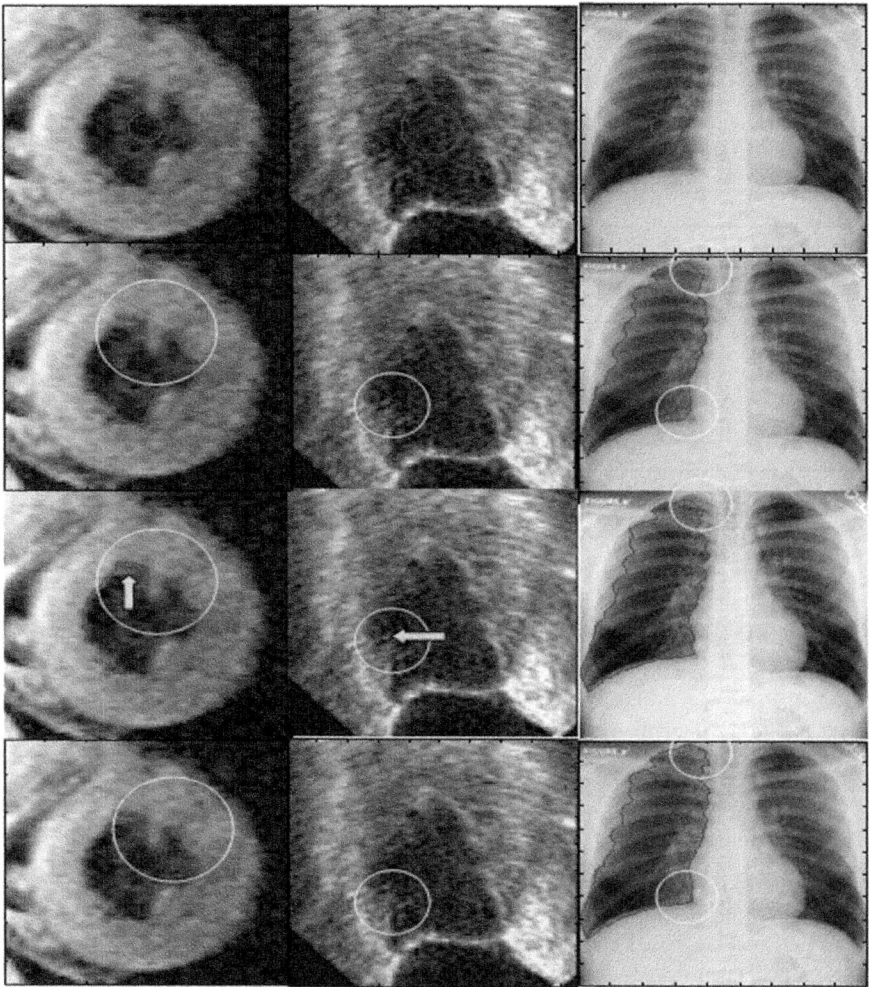

Fig. 1. Performance comparisons between the 3 models. Columns from left to right: magnetic resonance image of the left ventricles of a human heart; a noisy ultrasound image of the same organ but from a different view; a CT image of a pair of human lungs. The contours for segmentation are shown in red. Rows from top to bottom: the initial status of the contours; the segmentation results using the C-V model; the segmentation results using the LCV model; the bottom row is the segmentation results using our WC-V model. Note the difference in the regions highlighted by the yellow circles. The green arrows indicate the excessive segmentation of the tissue using the LCV model, indicating its vulnerability when LCV faces disturbances in local structures that are not located at tissue boundaries. The boundaries identified by our WC-V model are generally more accurate than those by other models.

Comparing the computation cost of the three models (Table 1) demonstrated that the WC-V model is much more efficient than other models. WC-V model cost only about half of the computer time that other models cost in segmentation of the MR and ultrasound images, and the WC-V model cost significantly less in segmentation of the

CT image (Table 1). To correctly segment the CT image of human lungs, the LCV required a relatively large local region. However, this enlargement significantly increased the computational cost (Table 1).

Table 1. Iterations and CPU time (in seconds) by three models. The WC-V model requires less iterations and less computational time than other models.

	Fig. 1(column 1)		Fig. 1(column 2)		Fig. 1(column 3)	
	136x132 pixels		95x93 pixels		219x179 pixels	
	Iterations	time(s)	Iterations	time(s)	Iterations	time(s)
C-V	523	22.35	353	12.10	870	61.51
LCV	594	36.87	284	17.06	702	356.64
WC-V	248	11.25	190	6.89	757	57.09

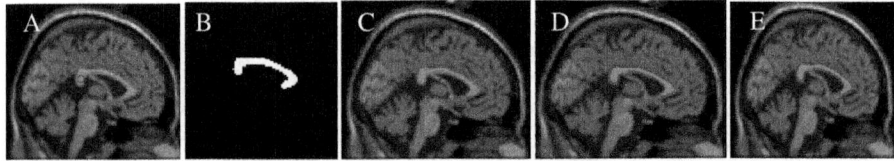

Fig. 2. Performance comparisons between the three models for segmentation of the CC of a human brain. (A) the initialization of the active contours; (B) the CC mask segmented manually by human experts; (C) The segmentation result using the C-V model; (D) The segmentation result using the LCV model; (E) The segmentation result using the WC-V model. The C-V model seems to be sensitive to the noise and non-uniformity levels, whereas the LCV model and WC-V model are not.

Table 2. A comparison of the average RSE of the segmentation results using the C-V, LCV and the WC-V models, based on 10 datasets of brain images. The WC-V model performs more efficient than other models.

(Noise, Non-Uniformity)	(0%, 0%)	(5%, 20%)	(9%, 40%)
C-V	34.4931	23.4094	28.4781
LCV	5.8803	6.3641	6.5377
WC-V	5.6165	5.6684	5.8985

5   Conclusion

We proposed a novel WC-V model for image segmentation by improving the traditional C-V model using a continuous weighting function. Because the classic C-V model treats all the point locations equally, it sometimes is unable to process correctly the medical images with intensity inhomogeneity, which is often the case in practice. In contrast, our WC-V model evaluates voxel contribution in the image based on its relative distance from the active contour, it therefore is able to segment images faster and more accurate than does the C-V model.

Although the WC-V model is based on the classical C-V model, our experiments using different image modalities demonstrated that the WC-V model outperformed the models of local segmentation [9] in terms of segmentation accuracy and computational costs, particularly for medical images with regional inhomogeneity of intensities.

Acknowledgement. NASARD Grant CU52051501, NIH Grant RO1MH09170, A Grant from SIMONS Foundation, NIDA Grant DA017820, NIBIB Grant 1R03EB008235-01A1, NIMH Grant 5R01MH082255-03, NIEHS Grant 1 R01 ES01557901 A2/ A2S109, Cina Natinal 985 Program, Shanghai Commission of Science and Technology Grant # 10440710200, supports from the Shanghai Key Laboratory of MR, and two grants from East China Normal University School of Psychology and Cognitive Neuroscience.

References

1. Kass, M., Witkin, A., Terzopoulos, D.: Snakes: active contour models. Int'l J. Comp. Vis. 1, 321–331 (1987)
2. Chan, T., Vese, L.: Active contour without edges. IEEE Trans. Imag. Proc. 10(2), 266–277 (2001)
3. Boykov, Y., Funka-Lea, G.: Graph cuts and efficient N-D image segmentation. IJCV 70, 109–131 (2006)
4. Comaniciu, D., Meer, P.: Mean shift: A robust approach toward feature space analysis. IEEE Trans. Pattern Anal. Machine Intell. 24(5), 603–618 (2002)
5. Caselles, V., Kimmel, R., Sapiro, G.: Geodesic active contours. Int'l J. Comp. Vis. 22(1), 61–79 (1997)
6. Kichenassamy, S., Kumar, A., Olver, P., Tannenbaum, A., Yezzi, A.: Gradient flows and geometric active contour models. In: Proc. 5th Int. Conf. Comp. Vis., pp. 810–815 (1995)
7. Osher, S., Tsai, R.: Level set methods and their applications in image science. Commun. Math. Sci. 1(4), 1–20 (2003)
8. Li, C., Kao, C., Gore, G., Ding, Z.: Minimization of region-scalable fitting energy for image segmentation. IEEE Trans. Imag. Proc. 17, 1940–1949 (2008)
9. Lankton, S., Tannenbaum, A.: Localizing Rigion-Based Active Contours. IEEE Trans. Image Process. 17(11), 2029–2039 (2008)
10. Zhang, K.H., Song, H.H., Zhang, L.: Active Contours Driven by Local Image Fitting Energy. Pattern Recognition 43(4), 1199–1206 (2010)
11. Krinidis, S., Chatzis, V.: Fuzzy Energy-Based Active Contours Image Processing. IEEE Trans. Imag. Proc. 18, 2747–2755 (2009)
12. Shi, Y., Karl, W.C.: A fast level set method without solving PDEs. In: IEEE International Conference on Acoustics, Speech, and Signal Processing, pp. 97–100 (2005)
13. Nilsson, B., Heyden, A.: A fast algorithm for level set-like active contours. Pattern Recogn. Lett. 24, 1331–1337 (2003)
14. Sethian, J.: Level Set Methods and Fast Marching Methods, 2nd edn. Springer, New York (1999)
15. http://en.wikipedia.org/wiki/Corpus_callosum
16. http://mouldy.bic.mni.mcgill.ca/brainweb/

Evaluation of Traumatic Brain Injury Patients Using a Shape-Constrained Deformable Model

Lyubomir Zagorchev, Carsten Meyer, Thomas Stehle, Reinhard Kneser,
Stewart Young, and Juergen Weese

Philips Research
lyubomir.zagorchev@philips.com

Abstract. Traumatic brain injury (TBI) is often associated with life long neurobehavioral effects in survivors. Imaging has historically supported the detection and acute management of life-threatening complications. However, in order to predict these long term consequences in the increasing number of individuals surviving TBI, there is an emerging need for structural neuroimaging biomarkers that would facilitate detection of milder injuries, allow recovery trajectory monitoring, and identify those at risk for poor functional outcome and disability. This paper presents a methodology capable of identifying such structural biomarkers in MR images of the brain. Results are presented demonstrating the quantitative accuracy of the approach with respect to (i) highly accurate annotations from expert tracers, (ii) an alternative segmentation method in FSL, and (iii) the ability to reproduce statistically significant differences in the volumes of specific structures between well-defined clinical cohorts (TBI vs age-matched healthy controls) in a retrospective analysis study.

Keywords: Neuro segmentation, brain model, traumatic brain injury.

1 Introduction

Traumatic brain injury (TBI) is a significant public health problem worldwide. Epidemiological studies vary but it is estimated that there are about 200 hospitalized cases of TBI each year per 100,000 population in Europe and North America. While Computed Tomography (CT) is the current modality of choice, in particular regarding identification of skull fractures, hemorrhages, contusions and edemas, Magnetic Resonance (MR) is superior in detecting cerebral and sub-cortical atrophy. It is thus suited for tracking structural volume changes in white/gray matter, long term outcome prediction, and tracking disease/recovery progression in follow-up studies [6].

Highly accurate quantification tools can address important outstanding issues, such as identifying the stage during injury progression at which structural changes can be reliably detected. One proposed approach for volumetric brain analysis involves the use of probabilistic atlases. In [5] a method that relies on Markov random fields to model local spatial relationships between neighboring structures in the context of a brain atlas was described. Other proposed

T. Liu et al. (Eds.): MBIA 2011, LNCS 7012, pp. 118–125, 2011.

approaches are based on learned statistical models of shape and intensity variation [8]. In [1] a comparison was presented of four methods for segmentation of sub-cortical brain structures, including approaches based on both atlases and statistical shape models, in which a multi-atlas approach exhibited the highest overall accuracy. That was, however, prohibitively computationally intensive for many clinical applications.

This work presents an approach for quantification of sub-cortical brain structure volumes, based on a shape-constrained deformable brain model. The approach is validated quantitatively with respect to both manual annotations created by expert tracers and an alternative method [5]. Then, the application of the approach in a retrospective clinical study is presented, using clinically well-defined cohorts including subjects with TBI and age-matched healthy controls. The method enables rapid, simultaneous segmentation of multiple structures, providing explicit descriptions of shape for all segmented structures, and provides a means to identify potential neuroimaging biomarkers.

2   Methods

Shape-constrained deformable surface models [10,4] combine the strengths of both deformable and active shape models by encoding a priori shape information while external forces guide the deformation and adapt the model to a target structure. A new shape-constrained deformable brain model that includes sub-cortical brain structures such as the amygdala, brainstem, caudate, cerebellum, corpus callosum, hippocampus, putamen, and thalamus, was developed for this work.

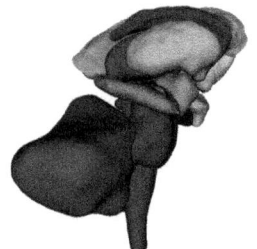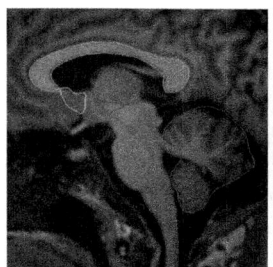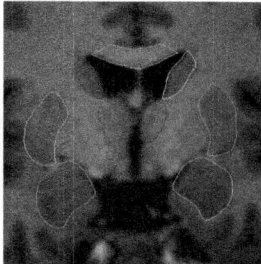

Fig. 1. Illustration of the shape-constrained deformable brain model

The model is represented by a triangular mesh which consists of V vertices and T triangles, an illustration is provided in Figure 1. During model creation, various properties describing the local image appearance and shape variation are extracted and learned from a set of training volumes and their corresponding ground truth data. The ground truth data represents highly accurate segmentations of the structures included in the model from a set of high resolution anatomical MR volumes (3T, T1-weighted, MPRAGE, 1x1x1.2 mm^3 voxel size).

The volumes in the training set were segmented manually by expert tracers using a software prototype for interactive manipulation of parametric spline contours. Corresponding boundary surfaces were recovered as triangular meshes. The mean mesh for each structure was obtained and all mean meshes were combined together, to define the geometry of the final model. Then, the surface meshes of each ground truth volume were resampled to contain the same number of vertices and triangles as the mean mesh. That enforces correspondence between triangles from the same mesh in different patients.

Every triangle in the model is associated with a feature function F. The goal of the feature function is to identify the optimal target position for a triangle by discriminating between different candidate positions according to an expected boundary appearance. The feature functions are selected and assigned to each triangle in the feature training step. A set of possible feature function candidates is evaluated in terms of accuracy with which the target points are detected in a simulated search. Object boundaries in general can be detected by projecting the image gradient ∇I onto the triangle normal $\mathbf{n}$ [9]. This suppresses the effect of edges (high gradients) which deviate from the expected surface orientation. Furthermore, gradients exceeding a certain threshold g_{max} can be damped, yielding:

$$G_{proj}(\mathbf{x}) = \pm(\mathbf{n} \cdot \nabla I(\mathbf{x})) \frac{g_{max}(g_{max} + ||\nabla I(\mathbf{x})||)}{g_{max}^2 + ||\nabla I(\mathbf{x})||^2} \tag{1}$$

where $\mathbf{x}$ represents the coordinates of a target point in the 3-D volume. The feature function can be made even more discriminative by encoding additional knowledge that can be used to reject edges if the local image properties violate some criteria as

$$F(\mathbf{x}) = \begin{cases} \pm G_{proj}(\mathbf{x}) \text{ if } Q_k \in [Min_k, Max_k] \text{ for all } Q_k \in S \\ 0 \qquad\qquad\qquad \text{otherwise} \end{cases} \tag{2}$$

where S is a set of image quantities Q_k and $[Min_k, Max_k]$ represents a range of allowed values learned from the training data. If at least one of the image quantities falls outside of the learned range, the edge will be rejected by setting the feature response to 0. The $\pm$ sign accounts for the expected transition of image intensities along the triangle normal (bright-to-dark or dark-to-bright). The quantities Q_k include the gray values on the both sides of the detected edge and the first and second order Taylor coefficient of the intensity values along the triangle normal.

The adaptation of the model to a volume is guided by the minimization of an energy term defined as a weighted sum of external and internal energies

$$E = E_{ext} + \alpha E_{int} \tag{3}$$

The external energy moves the mesh towards detected image boundaries while the internal energy penalizes deviation from a shape model. The parameter α acts as a weighting term that balances the effect of the two energies.

The adaptation is an iterative process that combines a boundary detection step with a deformation step. The boundary detection is accomplished by finding a target point x_i for mesh triangle i such that it maximizes the response of the associated feature function F along the normal of that triangle. The external energy then penalizes the squared distance between each triangle center c_i and the plane tangent to the detected boundary:

$$E_{ext} = \sum_{i=1}^{T} w_i \left(\frac{\nabla I(\mathbf{x}_i)}{||\nabla I(\mathbf{x}_i)||} \cdot (\mathbf{c}_i - \mathbf{x}_i) \right)^2 \tag{4}$$

The projection of $(\mathbf{c}_i - \mathbf{x}_i)$ onto the image gradient direction allows for sliding of the triangle along the detected image boundary. The weight w_i reflects the response of the feature function F and results in high values for reliably detected boundaries and low values for ill-defined boundaries. The internal energy penalizes the mesh for deviating from the mean shape during adaptation. The mean shape is derived from the ground truth data and can be augmented with shape variation modes obtained from a Principal Component Analysis (PCA) [3]. Alternatively, the mean mesh can be subdivided into K anatomical regions and the shape variation can be modeled with piecewise affine transformations $\mathcal{T}_K$; one assigned to each region K. The affine transformations allow for independent orientation and scaling of the individual regions. Smooth connection between regions is accomplished by a weighted linear combination of affine transformations:

$$\mathcal{T}_{\text{piecewise affine}}[\mathbf{v}_j] = \sum_{k=1}^{K} w_{j,k} \cdot \mathcal{T}_{\text{affine},k}[\mathbf{v}_j] \tag{5}$$

where $w_{j,k}$ are interpolation weights for vertex j, or $\mathbf{v}_j$, and $\sum_{k=1}^{K} w_{j,k} = 1$. Therefore, the internal energy is defined as:

$$E_{int} = \sum_{j=1}^{V} \sum_{l \in N(j)} \sum_{k=1}^{K} w_{j,k} \cdot ((\mathbf{v}_j - \mathbf{v}_l) - (\mathcal{T}_k[\mathbf{m}_j] - \mathcal{T}_k[\mathbf{m}_l]))^2 . \tag{6}$$

where $N(j)$ is the set of edge-connected neighbor vertices for vertex j, and $\mathbf{m}_j$ and $\mathbf{m}_l$ are the coordinates of vertices j and l in the mean mesh. As defined, the internal energy penalizes deviations in length and orientation for all edges between the mesh during adaptation and the shape model.

The described adaptation works well if the model is initialized relatively close to its target location. Robust, fully automatic segmentation of an arbitrary volume is accomplished by adding a number of additional image processing steps. First, the Generalized Hough Transform is applied to detect the approximate position of the model in the volume [2]. Then, an iterative global pose adaptation is performed by applying a global similarity transformation to all anatomical regions defined in the model. In the next step, individual affine transformations are assigned to each of the K anatomical mesh regions for a piecewise pose adaptation. The iterative application of boundary detection and piecewise mesh adaptation during this step results in a close alignment with the volume. Finally, when the model is already quite close to the anatomical structures in the volume, the deformable adaptation step described above further improves the alignment of the mesh vertex positions with the corresponding target structures.

3   Results

The adaptation of the model to a new volume is fully automatic. With the current version of the code, the computation time is less than 1 minute on an Intel Core2 Duo CPU T8300 at 2.4 GHz with 4Gb of RAM. It should also be noted that detailed speed optimizations have not been considered and that all brain structures are segmented simultaneously. Illustration of the segmentation of an arbitrary volume is shown in the Figure 1 above.

Quantitative evaluation of the accuracy of segmentation was performed using manually expert-traced ground truth data in a leave-one-out approach. A training set of 8 manually traced volumes with corresponding ground truth reference meshes was partitioned into two groups, one for training and one for validation. Seven volumes were used for training and one was left out for validation. Following that strategy, the same experiment was performed eight times, using different training and validation volumes at each round. Since the vertex correspondence between ground truth reference meshes and their counterparts in the model is preserved during adaptation, a reliable quantitative performance metric can be obtained. In this experiment, the distance between a triangle center and its corresponding closest point on the ground truth reference mesh was evaluated for all triangles. The mean and root-mean-squared (RMS) distances per structure were measured. It should be noted that the closest point to surface distance is not necessarily a symmetric measure in the most general case. Therefore, the above distances were measured twice: from the adapted model to ground truth reference meshes and vice versa. The averages of the two measurements were used to quantify the performance of the model. The first row in Figure 2 shows the average mean and RMS distance measures from all evaluation rounds. In addition, the volume of modeled brain structures after adaptation was compared with the volume of corresponding ground truth reference meshes. Thus, two other quantitative measures were obtained: the absolute volume difference between corresponding structures, and the Dice's coefficient. Both are shown on the second row in Figure 2.

In order to compare the performance of the shape-constrained deformable brain model with FSL [5], a set of 9 healthy control patients was imaged at two different time points and segmented with both FSL and the proposed method. Difference in volume per structure between the two time points was calculated and compared in order to assess the variability of results. Please note that healthy control patients should not exhibit any signs of brain structure atrophy, or volumetric changes, over a relatively short period of time. Qualitative visual comparisons and quantitative evaluation illustrated as the average relative difference of volume for all structures are shown in Figure 3. The examples indicate that our method provides improved consistency and reliability of results. Furthermore, FSL segments a volume one structure at a time, while the brain model segments

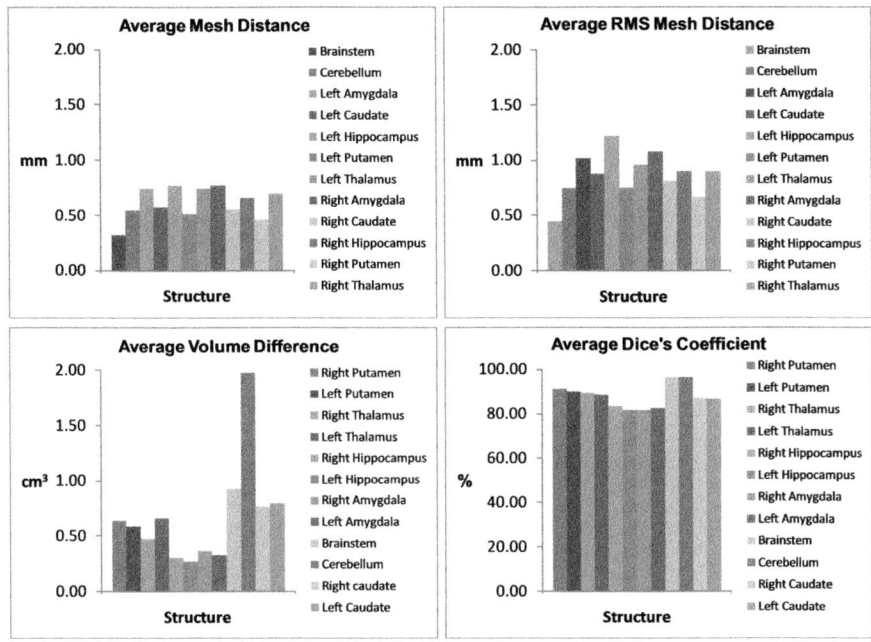

Fig. 2. Quantitative evaluation with respect to ground truth data

all brain structures simultaneously. That has two important implications: 1) our method prevents the intersection of neighboring structures during adaptation, and 2)provides a fully automatic segmentation that can be used by even an untrained user.

And finally, in an attempt to validate the sensitivity of the brain model for developing neuroimaging biomarkers for TBI, it was applied to the retrospective evaluation of a cohort of age-matched male subjects: healthy controls and individuals diagnosed with moderate TBI. Statistical analysis was used to assess the amount of detected volumetric changes. In particular, independent samples T-tests were performed to examine the significant difference between group means. The volume of all structures included in the model was measured in the control and TBI groups. Obtained measurements were grouped per structure and independent samples T-test was applied to each group. It should be noted that the volume of structures was not normalized to account for different head sizes. Previous work suggests that such correction removes true measurements' variance and may result in reduced reliability and artificially enhanced criterion validity [7]. In this evaluation, the group of control patients (n=16) was measured with the shape-constrained deformable brain model and results were compared with similar measurements from the age-matched group of moderate TBI patients(n=10). Significant bilateral volumetric difference in the putamen, thalamus, caudate, and brainstem was detected as illustrated in Figure 4.

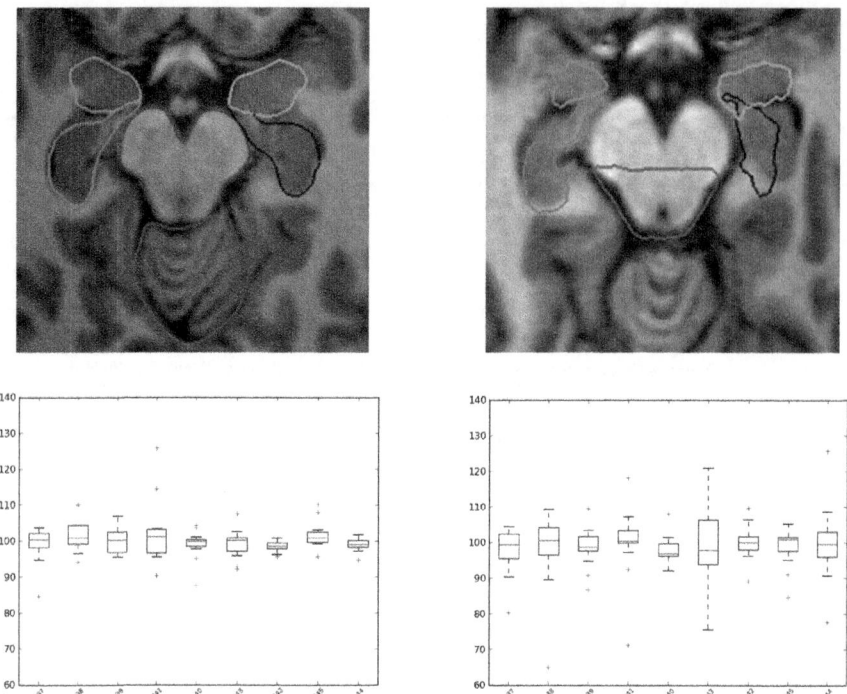

Fig. 3. Comparison between the brain model (left) and FSL (right). The horizontal axis of the charts shows the patient ID number while the vertical axis shows a Box-Whisker plot of the relative volume difference between the two time points for all structures.

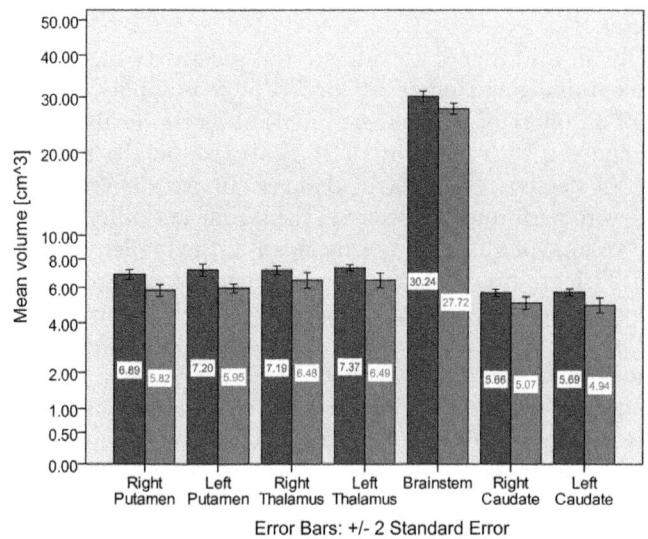

Fig. 4. Statistically significant differences detected between the control (blue) and TBI (green) groups (95% confidence interval, p values: .000,.000,.020,.001,.005,.006,.001)

4   Conclusion

The ability to have rapid and highly accurate evaluation of volume and shape of a large number of brain structures would allow for the development of novel imaging biomarkers that are needed in the diagnosis and monitoring of TBI. It would allow for tracking of measurements over time and their correlation with various functional modalities. The preliminary results presented in this work suggest that the shape-constrained deformable brain model has the necessary sensitivity to detect volumetric changes in affected individuals. It has the potential to greatly enhance our understanding of underlying disease mechanisms and their related clinical manifestation.

References

1. Babalola, K., Patenaude, B., Aljabar, P., Schnabel, J., Kennedy, D., Crum, W., Smith, S., Cootes, T., Jenkinson, M., Rueckert, D.: An evaluation of four automatic methods of segmenting the subcortical structures in the brain. Neuroimage 47(4), 1435–1447 (2009)
2. Ballard, D.: Generalizing the hough transform to detect arbitrary shapes. Pattern Recognition 13(2), 111–122 (1981)
3. Cootes, T., Taylor, C., Cooper, D., Graham, J., et al.: Active shape models-their training and application. Computer Vision and Image Understanding 61(1), 38–59 (1995)
4. Ecabert, O., Peters, J., Schramm, H., Lorenz, C., von Berg, J., Walker, M., Vembar, M., Olszewski, M., Subramanyan, K., Lavi, G., et al.: Automatic model-based segmentation of the heart in CT images. IEEE Transactions on Medical Imaging 27(9), 1189–1201 (2008)
5. Fischl, B., Salat, D., Busa, E., Albert, M., Dieterich, M., Haselgrove, C., van der Kouwe, A., Killiany, R., Kennedy, D., Klaveness, S., et al.: Whole brain segmentation automated labeling of neuroanatomical structures in the human brain. Neuron 33(3), 341–355 (2002)
6. Jorge, R., Robinson, R., Moser, D., Tateno, A., Crespo-Facorro, B., Arndt, S.: Major depression following traumatic brain injury. Archives of General Psychiatry 61(1), 42 (2004)
7. Mathalon, D., Sullivan, E., Rawles, J., Pfefferbaum, A.: Correction for head size in brain-imaging measurements. Psychiatry Research: Neuroimaging 50(2), 121–139 (1993)
8. Patenaude, B., Smith, S., Kennedy, D., Jenkinson, M.: Bayesian shape and appearance models. Tech. rep., TR07BP1, FMRIB Center, University of Oxford (2007)
9. Peters, J., Ecabert, O., Meyer, C., Kneser, R., Weese, J.: Optimizing boundary detection via simulated search with applications to multi-modal heart segmentation. Medical Image Analysis 14(1), 70 (2010)
10. Weese, J., Kaus, M.R., Lorenz, C., Lobregt, S., Truyen, R., Pekar, V.: Shape constrained deformable models for 3D medical image segmentation. In: Insana, M.F., Leahy, R.M. (eds.) IPMI 2001. LNCS, vol. 2082, pp. 380–387. Springer, Heidelberg (2001)

Human Brain Mapping with Conformal Geometry and Multivariate Tensor-Based Morphometry

Jie Shi[1], Paul M. Thompson[2], and Yalin Wang[1]

[1]School of Computing, Informatics and Decision Systems Engineering,
ASU, Tempe, AZ 85281, USA
[2]Lab. of Neuro Imaging, UCLA School of Medicine, Los Angeles, CA 90095, USA
jie.shi@asu.edu

Abstract. In this paper, we introduce theories and algorithms in conformal geometry, including Riemann surface, harmonic map, holomorphic 1-form, and Ricci flow, which play important roles in computational anatomy. In order to study the deformation of brain surfaces, we introduce the multivariate tensor-based morphometry (MTBM) method for statistical computing. For application, we introduce our system for detecting Alzheimer's Disease (AD) symptoms on hippocampal surfaces with an automated surface fluid registration method, which is based on surface conformal mapping and mutual information regularized image fluid registration. Since conformal mappings are diffeomorphic and the mutual information method is able to drive a diffeomorphic flow that is adjusted to enforce appropriate surface correspondences in the surface parameter domain, combining conformal and fluid mappings will generate 3D shape correspondences that are diffeomorphic. We also incorporate in the system a novel method to compute curvatures using surface conformal parameterization. Experimental results in ADNI baseline data diagnostic group difference and APOE4 effects show that our system has better performance than other similar work in the literature.

1 Introduction

Conformal structure is an intrinsic feature of a metric surface. All oriented surfaces have conformal structures. Many recent researches have used algorithms from conformal geometry for computational analysis of brain anatomy. For brain surface flattening [7] and brain surface parameterization research, Hurdal et al. [11] reported a discrete mapping approach that uses circle packings to produce "flattened" images of cortical surfaces on the sphere, the Euclidean plane, and the hyperbolic space. The maps obtained are quasi-conformal approximations of classical conformal maps. [2] implemented a finite element approximation for parameterizing brain surfaces via conformal mappings. Gu et al. [8] proposed a method to find a unique conformal mapping between any two genus zero manifolds by minimizing the harmonic energy of the map. The holomorphic 1-form based conformal parameterization [18] can conformally parameterize high genus surface with boundaries but the resulting mappings have singularities. The Ricci

T. Liu et al. (Eds.): MBIA 2011, LNCS 7012, pp. 126–134, 2011.
© Springer-Verlag Berlin Heidelberg 2011

flow method [17] can handle surfaces with complicated topologies (boundaries and landmarks) without singularities.

In general, in order to study the deformation of cortical surfaces, there exist two different approaches, deformation-based morphometry (DBM) [5] and tensor-based morphometry (TBM) [6]. One advantage of TBM for surface morphometry is that it can use the intrinsic Riemannian surface metric to characterize local changes. [12,20] proposed a new multivariate TBM framework for surface morphometry. MTBM computes statistics from the Riemannian metric tensors that retain the full information in the deformation tensor fields, thus is more powerful in detecting surface differences [20].

Using holomorphic 1-forms, a global conformal parameterization can be developed to conformally map a surface to a rectangular domain in the Euclidean plane. The mutual information (MI) method has been widely used to drive a diffeomorphic flow in image registration. By adjusting the mutual information method to enforce appropriate surface correspondences in the parameter domain, any scalar-valued signals defined on the surfaces can also be aligned using the same flow field. Conformal maps and fluid registration techniques can be combined to avoid having to define a large set of manually-defined landmarks. Since they generate diffeomorphic mappings, conformal and fluid mappings together could generate 3D shape correspondences that are diffeomorphic (i.e., smooth one-to-one correspondences). In [16], Wang et al. proposed an automated surface fluid registration method based on conformal mapping and mutual information regularized image fluid registration and applied it to register human faces and hippocampus. Here we develop a system based on this technique for studying hippocampus in Alzheimer's Disease and incorporate a novel method to compute surface curvatures as proposed in [13]. Our major contributions can be summarized as: (1). Introduction of a new stable method to compute surface curvatures. (2). An automated hippocampal surface segmentation and registration system validated in ADNI baseline data. (3). The system will be publicly available [21]. Last, although the current system finds applications in AD detection, it is a general method which may be applied to many other applications.

2   Theoretical Background

Here we briefly introduce some theories in conformal geometry. For details, we refer readers to [10] for algebraic topology and [9] for differential geometry.

2.1   Riemann Surface

Let S be a surface in $\mathbb{R}^3$ with an atlas $\{(U_\alpha, z_\alpha)\}$, where (U_α, z_α) is a coordinate chart defined on S. The atlas thus is a set of consistent charts with smooth transition functions between overlapping charts. Here $z_\alpha : U_\alpha \to \mathbb{C}$ maps an open set $U_\alpha \subset S$ to a complex plane $\mathbb{C}$. If on any chart (U_α, z_α) in the atlas, the *Riemannian metric* or the *first fundamental form* can be formulated as $ds^2 = \lambda(z_\alpha)^2 dz_\alpha d\bar{z}_\alpha$, and the transition maps $z_\beta \circ z_\alpha^{-1} : z_\alpha(U_\alpha \bigcap U_\beta) \to$

$z_\beta(U_\alpha \cap U_\beta)$ are holomorphic, the atlas could be called *conformal*. Given a conformal atlas, a chart is *compatible* with the atlas if adding this chart still generates a conformal atlas. A *conformal structure* is obtained by adding all possible compatible charts to a conformal atlas. A *Riemann surface* is a surface with a conformal structure. All metric surfaces are Riemann surfaces. Following the uniformization theorem [1], we can embed any Riemann surface onto one of the three canonical surfaces: the sphere $\mathbb{S}^2$ for genus zero surfaces with positive Euler numbers, the plane $\mathbb{E}^2$ for genus one surfaces with zero Euler numbers, and the hyperbolic space $\mathbb{H}^2$ for high genus surfaces with negative Euler numbers.

2.2   Harmonic Maps

For genus zero surfaces, the major algorithm to compute their conformal mapping is *harmonic maps*. Suppose S_1, S_2 are two metric surfaces embedded in $\mathbb{R}^3$. $\phi : S_1 \to S_2$ is a map from S_1 to S_2. The *harmonic energy*, which measures the stretching of ϕ, is defined as $E_\phi = \int_{S_1} \|\nabla \phi\|^2 dA$. A *harmonic map* is a map ϕ that minimizes the harmonic energy. It can be easily computed by the steepest descent algorithm:

$$\frac{d\phi}{dt} = -\Delta\phi \tag{1}$$

The normal component of the Laplacian $\Delta\phi$ is $\Delta\phi^\perp = < \Delta\phi, \mathbf{n}(\phi) > \mathbf{n}(\phi)$. If ϕ is a harmonic map, then we should have $\Delta\phi = \Delta\phi^\perp$. Then Eq. 1 can be solved as $\frac{d\phi}{dt} = -(\Delta\phi - \Delta\phi^\perp)$. Fig. 1 (a) shows an example of the harmonic map.

2.3   Holomorphic 1-Form and Slit Mapping

Let S be a surface embedded in $\mathbb{R}^3$ with induced Euclidean metric $\mathbf{g}$. S is covered by atlas $\{(U_\alpha, z_\alpha)\}$ and (x_α, y_α) is the local parameter on a chart. Suppose ω is a differential 1-form with the representation $f(x_\alpha, y_\alpha)dx_\alpha + g(x_\alpha, y_\alpha)dy_\alpha$. ω is a *closed 1-form* if on each parameter (x_α, y_α), $\frac{\partial f}{\partial y_\alpha} - \frac{\partial g}{\partial x_\alpha} = 0$. ω is an *exact 1-form* if it equals to the gradient of another function defined on S. An exact 1-form is also a closed 1-form. If a closed 1-form ω satisfies $\frac{\partial f}{\partial x_\alpha} + \frac{\partial g}{\partial y_\alpha} = 0$, then ω is a *harmonic 1-form*. A *holomorphic 1-form* is a complex differential form $\tau = \omega + \sqrt{-1}^*\omega$, where ω is a harmonic 1-form and $^*\omega = -g(x_\alpha, y_\alpha)dx_\alpha + f(x_\alpha, y_\alpha)dy_\alpha$ is the conjugate of ω, which is also a harmonic 1-form. Fig. 1 (b) shows an example of the holomorphic 1-form. Fix a point p_0 on the surface, for any point $p \in S$, let γ be an arbitrary path connecting p_0 and p, the mapping $\phi(p) = e^{\int_\gamma \tau}$ is called slit mapping. Fig. 1 (c) shows the result of slit mapping.

2.4   Ricci Flow

The Ricci flow is the process to deform a metric $\mathbf{g}(t)$ according to its induced Gaussian curvature $K(t)$, where t denotes the time parameter: $\frac{d\mathbf{g}(t)}{dt} = -K(t)\mathbf{g}(t)$. There is an analog between Ricci flow and the heat diffusion process. When Ricci flow converges, the metric $\mathbf{g}(t)$ at time t is conformal to the original metric and the Gaussian curvature is constant everywhere. Fig. 1 (d) and (e) show the results of the Euclidean and hyperbolic Ricci flow, respectively.

Harmonic En- ergy Minimization	Holomorphic 1-form	Circular Slitmap	Euclidean Ricci flow	Hyperbolic Ricci flow

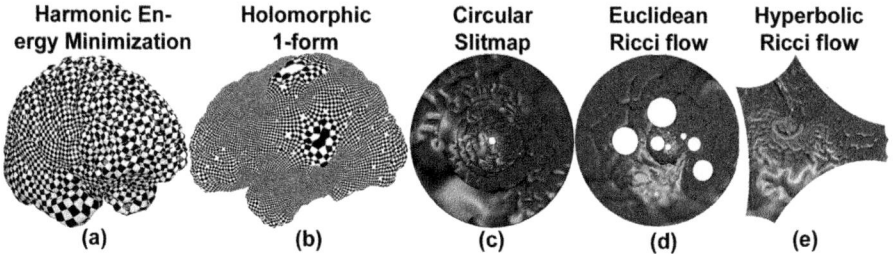

|(a)|(b)|(c)|(d)|(e)|

Fig. 1. Various conformal parameterization results

2.5   Multivariate Tensor Based Morphometry

Suppose $\phi : S_1 \rightarrow S_2$ is a map from surface S_1 to surface S_2. The derivative map of ϕ is the linear map between the tangent spaces, $d\phi : TM(p) \rightarrow TM(\phi(p))$, induced by the map ϕ, which also defines the Jacobian matrix of ϕ. Let J be the Jacobian matrix and define the deformation tensors as $S = (J^T J)^{\frac{1}{2}}$. Instead of analyzing shape change based on the eigenvalues of the deformation tensors, a new family of metrics, the "Log-Euclidean metrics" [3], which are computed by inverse of matrix exponential, are considered. Hotelling's T^2 test is applied on sets of values in the Log-Euclidean space of the deformation tensors. Given two groups of n-dimensional vectors $S_i, i = 1, ..., p, T_j = 1, ..., q$, let $\bar{S}$ and $\bar{T}$ be the means of the two groups and $\sum$ is the combined covariance matrix of the two groups. The Mahalanobis distance $M = (log\bar{S} - log\bar{T}) \sum^{-1} (log\bar{S} - \bar{T})$ is used to measure the group mean difference. For details of MTBM, we refer to [12,20].

3   Applications

Conformal geometry has broad applications in medical imaging, geometric modeling and many other fields. Recent years, we have applied it in brain surface conformal parameterization [17,18,19], brain surface registration [16], MRI-based biomarker detection with machine learning [22], and neonate brain study. In this section, we highlight an automated surface registration system based on the combination of surface conformal mapping and image fluid registration methods. Surface registration usually requires defining a lot of landmarks in order to align corresponding functional regions. Labeling features could be accurate but time-consuming. Here we show that surface conformal mapping could represent surface geometric features, thus avoiding the manual definition of landmarks.

For a general surface and its conformal mapping $\phi : S \rightarrow \mathbb{R}^2$, the conformal factor at a point p can be determined by the formulation: $\lambda(p) = \frac{\text{Area}(B_\epsilon(p))}{\text{Area}(\phi(B_\epsilon(p)))}$, where $B_\epsilon(p)$ is an open ball around p with a radius ϵ. The conformal factor λ encodes a lot of geometric information about the surface and can be used to compute curvatures and geodesic. In our system, we compute the surface mean curvatures only from the derivatives of the conformal parameterization as proposed in [13], instead of the three coordinate functions and the normal, which are generally more sensitive to digitization errors. Mathematically, the mean curvature is defined as:

$$H = \frac{1}{2\lambda}\text{sign}(\phi)|\Delta\phi|, \ \text{where sign}(\phi) = \frac{<\Delta\phi, \overrightarrow{N}>}{|\Delta\phi|} \qquad (2)$$

In this formulation of H, we need to use the surface normal $\overrightarrow{N}$ only when computing $\text{sign}(\phi)$, which takes the value 1 or -1. Thus, the surface normal does not need to be accurately estimated and still we can get more accurate mean curvatures. Using the Gauss and Codazzi equations, one can prove that the conformal factor and mean curvature uniquely determine a closed surface in $\mathbb{R}^3$, up to a rigid motion. We call them the *conformal representation* of the surface. Since conformal factor and mean curvature could represent important surface features and are intrinsic to the surface, they may be used for surface registration.

After computing intrinsic geometric features, we align surfaces in the parameter domain with a fluid registration technique.Using conformal mapping, we essentially convert the surface registration problem to an image registration problem. In [16], Wang et al. proposed an automated surface fluid registration method combining conformal mapping and image fluid registration. Since conformal mapping and MI regularized fluid registration generate diffeomorphic mappings, a diffeomorphic surface-to-surface mapping is then recovered that matches surfaces in 3D. In our system, we adopt their methods of conformal mapping and fluid registration. However, our system differs from theirs in the computation of surface features as introduced above. The new way to compute mean curvature is more stable and less sensitive to normal computation, thus gives better representation of the surface features for registration.

4   Experimental Results

We applied our surface registration system to study hippocampal surface morphometry in AD. In our study, we tested the system on the Alzheimer's Disease Neuroimaging Initiative (ADNI) baseline data (http://www.loni.ucla.edu/ADNI). The data contains 233 healthy controls, 410 subjects with mild cognitive impairment (MCI), and 200 patients with AD. The hippocampal surfaces were automatically segmented using FIRST (http://www.fmrib.ox.ac.uk/fsl/fsl/list.html). FIRST is an integrated registration and segmentation tool developed as part of the FSL library, which is written mainly by members of the Analysis Group, FMRIB, Oxford, UK. We also took FIRST's technique of registration for a comparison in our diagnostic group difference study. In the segmentation step, 1 subject in each group (AD, MCI, and control) failed probably due to the original images' resolution or contrast. We also manually occluded 1 subject from the control group and 2 subjects from the MCI group because of name duplication. For subjects with duplicated names, we retained the one which was the repeated scan. Thus 837 subjects were involved in all the experiments in this paper.

In our system, we left two holes at the front and back of the hippocampal surface, representing its anterior junction with the amygdala, and its posterior limit as it turns into the white matter of the fornix. The resulting structure can then be logically represented as an open boundary genus one surface, i.e., a cylinder. Then the surfaces were conformally mapped to a rectangle plane using holomorphic 1-forms.To better visualize the matching of surface features, we chose to encode surface features using a compound scalar function based on the local conformal factor and the mean curvature. After the cross-subject registration was computed with one target surface selected, we examined shape differences using the MTBM as introduced in Sec. 2.5.

4.1   Effects of APOE4 Genotype

In [14], Morra et.al. discussed that in healthy elderly subjects, presence of the Apolipoprotein E ϵ4 allele (APOE4) may be correlated with future development of AD. In order to investigate this correlation, the authors designed two experiments: (1) group difference between APOE4 carriers and non-carriers in all samples; (2) group difference between APOE4 carriers and non-carriers in subjects that have not developed AD, i.e., MCI and control groups. The experiments are aimed to determine if the APOE4 allele is linked with hippocampal atrophy in all subjects and in just the non-AD subjects, respectively. In [14], 400 subjects with 100 AD, 200 MCI, and 100 control subjects from ADNI baseline data were studied. However, no significance was reported in [14]. In our study, among the 837 subjects, 738 subjects have been diagnosed as APOE4 carriers or non-carriers, 566 of which are MCI or controls. Fig. 2 shows the significance maps for APOE4 effects. With MTBM, our system has been able to detect more significant areas compared with [14]. The significant p-values are 0.00044 for the all-sample experiment and 0.02073 for the non-AD experiment, respectively.

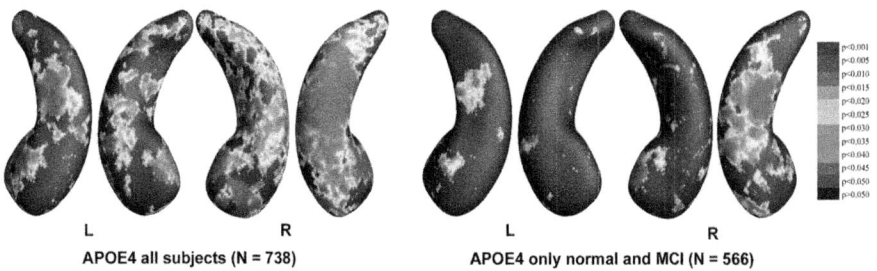

Fig. 2. Significance maps for APOE4 effects

In [15], Pievani et al. designed more systematic experiments to study APOE4 effects. We will study their findings in our ongoing work.

4.2   Diagnostic Group Differences

Fig. 3 illustrates the experimental results showing difference maps among the three diagnostic groups (AD, MCI and control). MCI is an intermediate stage between the expected cognitive decline of normal aging and the more pronounced decline of dementia. If MCI could be found and treated, the risk of AD will be significantly reduced. However, at MCI stage, changes in brain surface are not significant thus impose more difficulty on the detection. With MTBM, we can see that, in the three experiments, our system demonstrated better results than FIRST. Particularly, our system gave better MCI detection results when comparing with both AD and control subjects. In the experiment, all group difference p-maps were corrected using false discovery rate (FDR) [4]. The FDR method decides whether a threshold can be assigned to the statistical map that keeps the expected FDR below 5% (i.e., no more than 5% of the voxels are false positive findings). The CDF plots show the uncorrected p-values (as in a conventional FDR analysis). The x value at which the CDF plot intersects the $y = 20x$ line represents the highest statistical threshold that can be applied to the data, for which at most 5% false positives are expected in the map. The use of the $y = 20x$ line is related to the fact that significance is declared when the volume of suprathreshold statistics is more than 20 times that expected under the null hypothesis. Table 1 gives the FDR corrected p-values comparison.

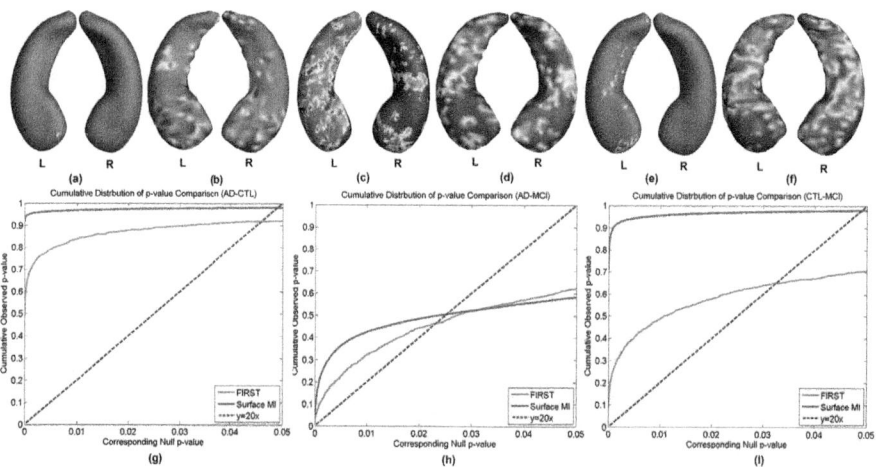

Fig. 3. Comparison of surface fluid registration and FIRST on map of local shape differences (p-values) between different diagnostic groups, based on the mutivariate TBM method with hippocampal surfaces in 199 AD, 407 MCI, and 231 control subjects which were automatically segmented by FIRST. (a), (c), (e) are our results on group difference between AD and control, AD and MCI, MCI and control, respectively. Similarly, (b), (d), (f) are results of FIRST on AD and control, AD and MCI, MCI and control, respectively. The p-map color scale is the same as Fig. 2. (g), (h), (i) are the CDF plots showing the comparisons.

Table 1. FDR corrected p-values on hippocampal surfaces

	Surface MI	FIRST
AD-CTL	0.0485	0.0419
AD-MCI	0.0215	0.0131
CTL-MCI	0.0483	0.0261

5   Conclusion and Future Work

This paper reviews some algorithms in conformal geometry and highlights an automated surface fluid registration system. Experiments on ADNI hippocampal dataset demonstrate our system's stronger statistical power than other work in the literature. Ongoing work is to apply this system to automatically map lateral ventricle enlargements in Alzheimers disease and those at risk.

References

1. Abikoff, W.: The uniformization theorem. The American Mathematical Monthly 88(8), 574–592 (1981)
2. Angenent, S., Haker, S., Tannenbaum, A.R., Kikinis, R.: Conformal geometry and brain flattening. In: Taylor, C., Colchester, A. (eds.) MICCAI 1999. LNCS, vol. 1679, pp. 271–278. Springer, Heidelberg (1999)
3. Arsigny, V., et al.: Log-Euclidean metrics for fast and simple calculus on diffusion tensors. Magn. Reson. Med. 56(2), 411–421 (2006)
4. Benjamini, Y., et al.: Controlling the false discovery rate: a practical and powerful approach to multiple testing. J. of the Royal Statistical Society 57, 289–300 (1995)
5. Chung, M.K., et al.: Deformation-based surface morphometry applied to gray matter deformation. NeuroImage 18(2), 198–213 (2003)
6. Chung, M.K., et al.: Tensor-based cortical surface morphometry via weighted spherical harmonic representation. IEEE Trans. Med. Imag. 27(8), 1143–1151 (2008)
7. Fischl, B., et al.: Cortical surface-based analysis II: Inflation, flattening, and a surface-based coordinate system. NeuroImage 9(2), 195–207 (1999)
8. Gu, X., et al.: Genus zero surface conformal mapping and its application to brain surface mapping. IEEE Trans. Med. Imag. 23(8), 949–958 (2004)
9. Guggenheimer, H.W.: Differential Geometry. Dover Publications, Mineola (1977)
10. Hatcher, A.: Algebraic Topology. Cambridge University Press, Cambridge (2006)
11. Hurdal, M.K., et al.: Cortical cartography using the discrete conformal approach of circle packings. NeuroImage 23, 119–128 (2004)
12. Lepore, N., Brun, C.A., Chiang, M.-C., Chou, Y.-Y., Dutton, R.A., Hayashi, K.M., Lopez, O.L., Aizenstein, H.J., Toga, A.W., Becker, J.T., Thompson, P.M.: Multivariate statistics of the jacobian matrices in tensor based morphometry and their application to HIV/AIDS. In: Larsen, R., Nielsen, M., Sporring, J. (eds.) MICCAI 2006. LNCS, vol. 4190, pp. 191–198. Springer, Heidelberg (2006)
13. Lui, L.M., et al.: Computation of curvatures using conformal parameterization. Communications in Information and Systems 8(1), 1–16 (2008)

14. Morra, J.H., et al.: Automated 3D mapping of hippocampal atrophy and its clinical correlates in 400 subjects with Alzheimer's disease, mild cognitive impairment, and elderly controls. Human Brain Mapping 30(9), 2766–2788 (2009)
15. Pievani, M., et al.: APOE4 is associated with greater atrophy of the hippocampal formation in Alzheimer's disease. NeuroImage 55, 909–919 (2011)
16. Wang, Y., et al.: Mutual information-based 3D surface matching with applications to face recognition and brain mapping. In: Proc. Intl Conf. Computer Vision, pp. 527–534 (2005)
17. Wang, Y., Gu, X., Chan, T.F., Thompson, P.M., Yau, S.-T.: Brain surface conformal parameterization with algebraic functions. In: Larsen, R., Nielsen, M., Sporring, J. (eds.) MICCAI 2006. LNCS, vol. 4191, pp. 946–954. Springer, Heidelberg (2006)
18. Wang, Y., et al.: Brain surface conformal parameterization using Riemann surface structure. IEEE Trans. Med. Imag. 26(6), 853–865 (2007)
19. Wang, Y., Gu, X., Chan, T.F., Thompson, P.M., Yau, S.-T.: Conformal slit mapping and its applications to brain surface parameterization. In: Metaxas, D., Axel, L., Fichtinger, G., Székely, G. (eds.) MICCAI 2008, Part I. LNCS, vol. 5241, pp. 585–593. Springer, Heidelberg (2008)
20. Wang, Y., Chan, T.F., Toga, A.W., Thompson, P.M.: Multivariate tensor-based brain anatomical surface morphometry via holomorphic one-forms. In: Yang, G.-Z., Hawkes, D., Rueckert, D., Noble, A., Taylor, C. (eds.) MICCAI 2009. LNCS, vol. 5761, pp. 337–344. Springer, Heidelberg (2009)
21. Wang, Y.: Multivariate tensor-based subcortical morphometry system (2011), http://gsl.lab.asu.edu/conformal.htm
22. Wang, Y., et al.: MRI-based biomarker detection using conformal slit maps and machine learning. In: 16th Annual Meeting of the Organization for Human Brain Mapping (2010)

Information-Theoretic Multi-modal Image Registration Based on the Improved Fast Gauss Transform: Application to Brain Images

Žiga Špiclin, Boštjan Likar, and Franjo Pernuš

Faculty of Electrical Engineering, Laboratory of Imaging Technologies,
University of Ljubljana, Tržaška 25, 1000 Ljubljana, Slovenia
{ziga.spiclin,bostjan.likar,franjo.pernus}@fe.uni-lj.si

Abstract. Performances of multi-modality image registration methods that are based on information-theoretic registration criteria crucially depend on the specific computational implementation. We proposed a new implementation based on the improved fast Gauss transform so as to estimate, from all available intensity samples, the intensity density functions needed to compute the information-theoretic criteria. The proposed and several other state-of-the-art implementations were tested and compared in 3-D rigid-body registration of multi-modal brain volumes. Experimental results indicate that the proposed implementation achieves the most consistent spatial alignment of brain volumes at a subpixel accuracy.

Keywords: image registration, multi-modality, Gauss transform, joint entropy, mutual information, brain.

1 Introduction

Understanding and diagnosis of the human brain have improved significantly since the introduction of multi-modality imaging in the medical workflow. For example, complementary insight into patient's anatomy and/or function is offered by computed tomography (CT), magnetic resonance (MR) and position emission tomography (PET) images. However, it is not an easy task for a human operator to routinely process a huge amount of multi-modality image data. Fortunately, various tasks can be simplified by advanced image visualization or can even be automated through computational image analysis. To use these computational tools, the multi-modality images first need to be spatially aligned, which is a task carried out by image registration methods.

Aligning two multi-modal images presents a difficult image registration problem, since the image intensities may not be directly comparable and, thus, the corresponding image structures cannot be easily detected. The most successful multi-modal image registration methods are based on the information-theoretic criteria [11,2,1,13] that try to evaluate the statistical dependence between the co-occurring image intensities. The key component of these criteria is the computation of the joint density function (JDF) that, together with the specific

T. Liu et al. (Eds.): MBIA 2011, LNCS 7012, pp. 135–142, 2011.

implementation of a particular information-theoretic criterion, crucially defines the performance of image registration method [4].

Information-theoretic criterion that follows directly from the JDF is the joint entropy (JE) [7,3]. Robustness of JE can be improved by mutual information (MI) and its normalized variants [11,2,8,13]. Viola [11] implemented MI, in which JDF was modeled by a kernel density method, however, this approach resulted in a high computational complexity proportional to the squared number of intensity samples (pixels). Therefore, only stochastic estimates of MI were computationally tractable for registering large 3-D images. Due to the stochastic nature of such MI estimates, the accuracy and especially the robustness of a registration method may be compromised. Computing the intensity histograms [2,8,13] is the most popular and highly efficient approach to estimating the JDF. However, the heuristic space partitioning in the construction of the intensity histogram raises several issues, i.e. high sensitivity to interpolation artifacts [2,10] and the problem of selecting a suitable noise-resistant (quasi-global) optimization method [4]. Instead of the heuristic space partitioning, Orchard and Mann [3] used the Gaussian mixture model (GMM) to cluster the co-occurring image intensities. They maximized the log-likelihood of GMM, which is equivalent to minimizing the JE, as the GMM in their approach actually represents the JDF. A problem with the GMM-based JDF is that the number of modes needs to be correctly specified, a parameter usually not known in advance. Another popular information-theoretic criterion is Rényi entropy that can be directly estimated by using minimal spanning trees (MST) [1,6]. A MST connects by a shortest overall path all the co-occurring image intensities that span the JDF. The main drawback of the MST approach is its sensitivity to bad initialization [6].

In this paper, we propose a new implementation of JE and MI criteria based on the approach by Viola [11], but in which the JDF is estimated from all intensity samples, achieved by using the improved fast Gauss transform (IFGT) [5]. We performed 3-D rigid-body registration of multi-modal brain volumes to test the proposed IFGT-based implementation and compare it to several state-of-the-art implementations [2,6,3]. The results indicate that higher registration accuracy can be achieved by the IFGT-based registration method and that the proposed implementation does not require case-specific parameter tuning.

2   The IFGT-Based Image Registration Method

Let $u_i = u(x_i)$ and $v_i = v(\mathcal{S}(x_i))$ be the intensities of the reference and the floating image, respectively, where $\mathcal{S}(x) : \mathbb{R}^d \to \mathbb{R}^d$ is a spatial coordinate mapping and where $x_i \in \Omega$ are lexicographically ordered spatial coordinates for $i = 1, \ldots, N$ in the overlapping spatial domain Ω of the two images. Commonly, the spatial coordinate mapping $\mathcal{S}(x)$ is a function of some parameters θ, i.e. $\mathcal{S}(x) = f(x, \theta)$ and the floating image intensities are dependent on θ, noted as v_i^θ. Intensity pairs in Ω can be compactly denoted as $z_i^\theta = [u_i, v_i^\theta]^{\mathrm{T}}$. The task now is to find the optimal parameters $\widehat{\theta}$ that optimize a criterion $\mathcal{C}(\theta)$, which measures the degree of spatial alignment between images u and v^θ.

For multi-modal image registration, the most widely applied criterion is the MI [4]. For images u and v^θ the MI is computed as:

$$\mathcal{C}_{\mathrm{MI}}(\theta) = H(u) + H(v^\theta) - H(z^\theta) , \qquad (1)$$

where $H(\,\cdot\,)$ are the entropy terms. The first two terms represent the entropy of the intensity distribution of each of the images, while the last term represents the entropy of the JDF of the intensity pairs z^θ. Entropy of a sample distribution of z is computed as $H(z) = -\sum_{i=1}^{N} p(z_i) \log p(z_i)$. Evaluating the entropy terms in Eq. (1) requires that the underlying continuous density functions $p(z)$ are accurately estimated based on the given discrete image intensity values.

2.1 Evaluating Entropy via Kernel Density Estimation

We will estimate the true density functions $p(z)$ by the kernel density method using a Gaussian kernel $G_\psi(z) = c_\psi \exp(-\frac{1}{2} z^\mathrm{T} \psi^{-1} z)$ as follows

$$p(z) \approx p^*(z) = \frac{1}{N} \sum_{j=1}^{N} G_\psi(z - z_j) , \qquad (2)$$

where ψ is the covariance of the Gaussian. Based on $p^*(z)$ the entropy can be approximately evaluated by a sample mean $H^*(z) = -1/N_k \sum_k \log p^*(z_k)$ [11]. By inserting Eq. (2) in the sample mean, the entropy estimate becomes

$$H^*(z) = -\frac{1}{N} \sum_{i=1}^{N} \log \frac{1}{N} \sum_{j=1}^{N} G_\psi(z_i - z_j) . \qquad (3)$$

Equation (3) represents the fundamental result proposed by Viola [11] that allows us to compute the analytical expression for the entropy gradient and then use it for entropy minimization.

2.2 Gradient-Based Entropy Minimization

We derive here a closed-form iteration step for minimizing the entropy expression in Eq. (3) for the purpose of registering two images u and v^θ. Recall that $z^\theta = [u\, v^\theta]^\mathrm{T}$, thus, we will show the expressions for minimizing $H^*(z^\theta)$ in Eq. (1), while similar expressions are also obtained for minimizing $H^*(v^\theta)$. The derivative of $H^*(z^\theta)$ with respect to θ is

$$\nabla_\theta H^*(z) = \frac{1}{N} \sum_{i=1}^{N} \sum_{j=1}^{N} W_\psi(z_i^\theta, z_j^\theta)\, \sigma_v^{-2}\, \tilde{v}_{ij}^\theta\, (\nabla_\theta \tilde{v}_{ij}^\theta) , \qquad (4)$$

where $\tilde{v}_{ij}^\theta = v_i^\theta - v_j^\theta$ and

$$W_\psi(z_i^\theta, z_j^\theta) = \frac{G_\psi(z_i^\theta - z_j^\theta)}{\sum_{k=1}^{N} G_\psi(z_i^\theta - z_k^\theta)} . \qquad (5)$$

Note that diagonal covariance is assumed as $\psi = \mathrm{diag}([\sigma_u^2 \, \sigma_v^2])$. A closed-form iteration step is obtained by setting $\nabla_\theta H^*(z^\theta) \to \mathbf{0}$ and using a linear approximation $\tilde{v}_{ij}^{\theta + \delta\theta} = \tilde{v}_{ij}^\theta + (\nabla_\theta \tilde{v}_{ij}^\theta)^{\mathrm{T}} \, \delta\theta$ in Eq. (4). This yields

$$\left[\sum_{i=1}^{N} \sum_{j=1}^{N} W_\psi(z_i^\theta, z_j^\theta) \, \sigma_v^{-2} \, (\nabla_\theta \, \tilde{v}_{ij}^\theta)(\nabla_\theta \, \tilde{v}_{ij}^\theta)^{\mathrm{T}} \right] \delta\theta =$$

$$-\left[\sum_{i=1}^{N} \sum_{j=1}^{N} W_\psi(z_i^\theta, z_j^\theta) \, \sigma_v^{-2} \, \tilde{v}_{ij}^\theta \, (\nabla_\theta \, \tilde{v}_{ij}^\theta) \right], \qquad (6)$$

or $A \, \delta\theta = b$, where A is a $P \times P$ matrix and b is a $P \times 1$ vector and P is the number of parameters in θ. By solving the linear system in Eq. (6) for $\delta\theta$ the parameters are updated as $\theta^l = \theta^{l-1} + \delta\theta$ in the lth iteration step.

2.3   Applying IFGT in the Gradient-Based Entropy Minimization

Expressions in Eq. (6) need to be evaluated for each pair (z_i^θ, z_j^θ), i.e. the computational complexity is proportional to $\mathcal{O}(N^2)$, which is usually prohibitively expensive in real registration cases. However, if we consider the sum over j's as a weighted sum of Gaussians, then the IFGT method [5] can be used to significantly speed up the computations to $\mathcal{O}(pN)$ with $p \ll N$. The IFGT proceeds by 1) dividing the samples $z_j^\theta \in \Omega$ into K clusters S_k, 2) computing the coefficients of multivariate Taylor series expansion of $z_j^\theta \in S_k$ about cluster centers μ_k as

$$C_\alpha^k(Q) = c_\alpha \sum_{x_j \in S_k} Q_j \otimes G_\psi(z_j^\theta - \mu_k) \left[\psi^{-1}(z_j^\theta - \mu_k) \right]^\alpha, \qquad (7)$$

where Q_j denotes a weight matrix, $\otimes$ the outer product and α the multi-indices of polynomial powers up to total degree $|\alpha|$. Final step 3) is to evaluate the Taylor series for z_i^θ [5]. The speedup is achieved by truncating the Taylor series in Eq. (7) for terms beyond total degree $|\alpha| \le p$ and by ignoring the influence of $G_\psi(z)$ for $\|r_i^k\| > \rho_\psi$, where $r_i^k = z_i^\theta - \mu_k$.

We used K-center algorithm to get K clusters S_k and computed the p-truncated Taylor series for $Q_j \otimes W_\psi(z_i^\theta, z_j^\theta)$ using Eq. (7). To get the linear system of the closed-form iteration step in Eq. (6), we evaluated the following expressions

$$L_i = D_{ii}^\theta - \sum_{\substack{\|r_i^k\| \le \rho_\psi \\ |\alpha| < p}} \left[C_\alpha^k(D_{jj}^\theta) - e_i^\theta \, C_\alpha^k(h_j^\theta)^{\mathrm{T}} - C_\alpha^k(h_j^\theta) \, (h_i^\theta)^{\mathrm{T}} \right] R_{\psi,\alpha}(r_i^k), \qquad (8)$$

$$m_i = g_{ii}^\theta - \sum_{\substack{\|r_i^k\| \le \rho_\psi \\ |\alpha| < p}} \left[C_\alpha^k(g_{jj}^\theta) - v_i^\theta \, C_\alpha^k(h_j^\theta) - h_i^\theta \, C_\alpha^k(v_j^\theta) \right] R_{\psi,\alpha}(r_i^k), \qquad (9)$$

$$n_i = \sum_{\substack{\|r_i^k\| \le \rho_\psi \\ |\alpha| < p}} C_\alpha^k(1) \, R_{\psi,\alpha}(r_i^k), \qquad (10)$$

where $D_{ij}^\theta = (\nabla_\theta v_i^\theta)(\nabla_\theta v_j^\theta)^{\mathrm{T}}$, $g_{ij}^\theta = v_i^\theta(\nabla_\theta v_j^\theta)$, $h_j^\theta = \nabla_\theta v_j^\theta$ and $R_{\psi,\alpha}(r_i^k) = G_\psi(r_i^k)\left[\psi^{-1}r_i^k\right]^\alpha$. Expressions in square brackets were obtained by expanding $\tilde{v}_{ij}^\theta$ in Eq. (6). By $A = \sigma_v^{-2}\sum_{i=1}^N L_i/n_i$ and $b = -\sigma_v^{-2}\sum_{i=1}^N m_i/n_i$ we obtain the linear system for the closed-form iteration step presented in Sec. 2.2.

Bandwidth Selection. The most important free parameters of the proposed IFGT-based method are the bandwidths σ_u and σ_v in the covariance matrix ψ. Since the bandwidths must be well tuned to the underlying intensity distributions, setting the bandwidths can be difficult in real registration tasks. To determine the bandwidth lower bound we used the oversmoothing principle [9]

$$\lfloor\psi\rfloor = \left[\frac{2^{-d}(d+8)^{(d+6)/2}}{16N\Gamma(\frac{d+8}{2})(d+2)}\right]^{2/(d+4)}\hat{\Sigma}, \tag{11}$$

where $\hat{\Sigma}$ is the diagonal sample covariance computed for z_i^θ over $\forall x_i \in \Omega$. The actual bandwidths were selected as $\psi = \lambda\lfloor\psi\rfloor$ for $\lambda \geq 1$.

Mutual Information. The derivations in Eqs. (4–10) hold for minimizing a single entropy term. To compute the gradient of MI in Eq. (1) we evaluate Eqs. (8–10) for $\nabla_\theta H(v^\theta)$ and $\nabla_\theta H(z^\theta)$ to obtain the matrices A_v, b_v and A_z, b_z, respectively. Then, by $A = A_v - A_z$ and $b = b_v - b_z$ we obtain the linear system for the closed-form iteration step.

3   Image Registration Experiments

Performance tests were carried out for the task of 3-D rigid-body registration of brain volumes, obtained from the training set of the Retrospective Image Registration Evaluation (RIRE) project [12]. The brain volumes in the training set, i.e. a CT, PET and three PD-, T1- and T2-weighted MR volumes, were first registered by a supplied gold standard registration and then rescaled and zero padded to $80 \times 80 \times 32$ isotropic voxels. To test the registration methods, a series of ten trial displacements were generated by combining three translations and three rotations, chosen randomly from the range [-5, 5] pixels and degrees, respectively. The trial displacements were applied to each pair of volumes prior to executing the registration methods. Given that five 3-D medical volumes are in the RIRE training set, there are ten different volume pairs that can be registered. Thus, a total of one hundred registrations were executed for each tested method. Execution times were also recorded.

The proposed IFGT-based method was tested for two popular image registration criteria, namely the joint entropy ($\mathcal{C}_{\mathrm{JE}}^{\mathrm{IFGT}}$) and the mutual information ($\mathcal{C}_{\mathrm{MI}}^{\mathrm{IFGT}}$). Besides the proposed IFGT-based method, we tested and compared the histogram-based MI ($\mathcal{C}_{\mathrm{MI}}^{\mathrm{HIST}}$) [2], the GMM-based ensemble clustering method [3] that implements a variant of the JE criterion ($\mathcal{C}_{\mathrm{JE}}^{\mathrm{GMM}}$) and the MST-based method [6] that computes the α–Rényi entropy ($\mathcal{C}_{\alpha-\mathrm{E}}^{\mathrm{GMM}}$). Histogram-, GMM- and the IFGT-based methods were implemented in Matlab/MEX. The codes

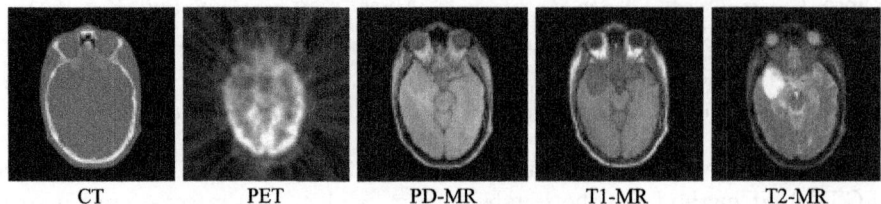

Fig. 1. Axial slices taken from the training set of the 3-D RIRE medical volumes, which were used to test the 3-D rigid-body registration methods

for the MST-based method were obtained from the author's website [6]. In the histogram-based method, the number of bins was set to $\sqrt{N}$, while the GMM-based method used $K = 6$ components to model the JDF. The MST-based method was initialized with default parameters ($\gamma = 1.9$, $\alpha = 0.5$). In the proposed IFGT-based method, the covariance scale factor λ was set to 5, while K, p and ρ_ψ were chosen automatically so that the density estimation error was $\epsilon < 0.001$ [5]. All image pairs were first registered at 50% of the original image resolution, then, the computed parameters were used as an initial guess for the registration at the original image resolution.

3.1 Results

The computed spatial coordinate mappings, as output by the registration methods, were compared to the gold standard ones. *Registration error* was defined as the average pixel coordinate displacement from its true (gold standard) position, computed over all pixels used in the registration ($\forall x_i \in \Omega$). The accuracy of the registration methods was measured by the *average registration error* computed over ten trial registrations for each image pair.

Registration Accuracy. The obtained registration accuracies for all tested methods are shown in Table 1. The proposed IFGT-based implementation of the MI achieved (on average) a subpixel accuracy of about 0.86 pixels, which was considerably more accurate than other tested state-of-the-art implementations based on the intensity histogram (1.59), the GMM (2.60) or the MST (2.32).

Execution Times. The average execution times for the histogram-, GMM- and MST-based implementations were 24, 39 and 0.67 seconds, respectively. For the proposed IFGT-based implementation the average execution times were 89 seconds for JE and 100 seconds for the MI criterion.

4   Discussion

Performances of multi-modal image registration methods based on information-theoretic registration criteria crucially depend on its computational implementation [4]. We proposed a new implementation of the information-theoretic criteria

Table 1. Average registration errors in pixels computed for a series of ten trial registrations of each pair of 3-D RIRE medical volumes for different variants and implementations of the information-theoretic criteria (cf. Sec. 3). The best result in each column is marked in bold. The initial average registration error was 5.03 pixels.

Method	CT-PET	CT-PD	CT-T1	CT-T2	PET-PD	PET-T1	PET-T2	PD-T1	PD-T2	T1-T2	Mean
C_{MI}^{HIST}	2.25	1.64	0.72	3.14	3.06	**1.22**	1.80	0.82	0.80	0.47	1.59
C_{JE}^{GMM}	**0.75**	8.58	0.80	5.47	1.55	3.49	4.79	**0.17**	0.16	**0.27**	2.60
$C_{\alpha-E}^{MST}$	1.43	0.90	1.25	2.34	2.47	5.37	3.17	0.82	1.85	3.63	2.32
C_{JE}^{IFGT}	0.98	0.44	0.28	**1.42**	0.95	1.69	2.36	0.25	0.15	2.27	1.08
C_{MI}^{IFGT}	1.09	**0.42**	**0.27**	1.59	**0.88**	1.28	**1.42**	0.27	**0.14**	1.26	**0.86**

based on the improved fast Gauss transform (IFGT) [5]. IFGT is used to estimate, from all available intensity samples, the intensity density functions that are needed to compute the information-theoretic criteria. The proposed and several other state-of-the-art implementations or methods [2,6,3] were tested and compared in 3-D rigid-body registration of multi-modal brain volumes. The results indicate that at only a slightly higher computational cost the proposed method achieves superior registration accuracy among the tested methods.

Registration methods should achieve optimal performances without a dedicated tuning of its characteristic parameters to the specific registration task. Therefore, during our registration experiments the above-specified parameter values (see Sec. 3) of the tested methods were held fixed so as to observe the sensitivity of the tested methods for different combinations of multi-modal image pairs. Registration accuracy for the GMM-based method was excellent in CT-PET and MR-MR registrations, but dropped significantly in CT-MR and PET-MR registrations (see Table 1). Since for most of CT-MR and PET-MR image pairs the GMM-based method failed completely, the GMM component number K might need to be tuned individually for each image pair to achieve optimal performance. The registration accuracy of MST-based method failed only in one CT-T1 registration, while overall it seems to produce a somehow biased, inaccurate registrations. Similar conclusions hold for the histogram-based implementation of MI, especially in the case of image pairs including CT and in PET-PD registration. The proposed IFGT-based methods performed slightly worse for some of the image pairs including the MR-T2 image (see Table 1), owing to two misregistered image pairs out of ten trials. However, among the tested methods the IFGT-based method produced the most consistent and the most accurate image pair registrations.

Computational complexity of tested methods is $\mathcal{O}(N)$ for the histogram-based, $\mathcal{O}(N \log N)$ for the MST-based, $\mathcal{O}(K N P^2 D^3)$ for the GMM-based and $\mathcal{O}(p N P^2 D^3)$ for the IFGT-based method. The GMM- and the IFGT-based methods have similar computational complexity because of the similar form of the entropy minimization step (Sec. 2.2). Due to the aggressive random sub-sampling scheme (1% of N) the MST-based method was suprisingly fast, but relatively inaccurate. To reduce execution time of the IFGT-based method we could implement a similar random subsampling scheme, but we believe it might compromise the registration accuracy. A better strategy would be to lower the total degree p, controlled by the approximation error ϵ, or taking high value of λ to speed up convergence from the initial position and, then, progressively lowering λ to avoid oversmoothing the density estimates as the registration progresses.

The proposed IFGT-based method achieves superior registration accuracy among the tested state-of-the-art information-theoretic multi-modality image registration methods. Higher accuracy comes at a higher computational cost, however, some viable solutions were proposed to tackle this issue. Moreover, the proposed IFGT-based method produced the most consistent registrations without tuning its parameters (λ and ϵ) specifically to each of the multi-modal image pairs tested in the registration experiments.

Acknowledgments. Supported by the Ministry of Higher Education, Science and Technology, Republic of Slovenia, under grants L2-2023, J2-2246, P2-0232.

References

1. Ma, B., Hero, A., Gorman, J., Michel, O.: Image registration with minimum spanning tree algorithm. In: Proceeding of the IEEE International Conference on Image Processing, vol. 1, pp. 481–484 (2000)
2. Maes, F., Collignon, A., Vadermeulen, D., Marchal, G., Suetens, P.: Multimodality image registration by maximization of mutual information. IEEE T. Med. Imag. 16(2), 187–198 (1997)
3. Orchard, J., Mann, R.: Registering a multisensor ensemble of images. IEEE T. Image Process. 19(5), 1236–1247 (2010)
4. Pluim, J.P.W., Maintz, J.B.A., Viergever, M.A.: Mutual-information-based registration of medical images: a survey. IEEE T. Med. Imag. 22(8), 986–1004 (2003)
5. Raykar, V.C., Duraiswami, R., Zhao, L.H.: Fast Computation of Kernel Estimators. J. Comput. Graph. Stat. 19(1), 205–220 (2010)
6. Sabuncu, M.R., Ramadge, P.: Using spanning graphs for efficient image registration. IEEE T. Image Process. 17(5), 788–797 (2008)
7. Studholme, C., Cardenas, V.: A template free approach to volumetric spatial normalization of brain anatomy. Pattern Recogn. Lett. 25(10), 1191–1202 (2004)
8. Studholme, C., Hill, D.L.G., Hawkes, D.J.: An overlap invariant entropy measure of 3D medical image alignment. Pattern Recogn. 32(1), 71–86 (1999)
9. Terrell, G.R.: The Maximal Smoothing Principle in Density Estimation. J. Amer. Statistical Assoc. 85(410), 470–477 (1990)
10. Thevenaz, P., Unser, M.: Optimization of mutual information for multiresolution image registration. IEEE T. Image Process. 9(12), 2083–2099 (2000)
11. Viola, P.A.: Alignment by maximization of mutual information, Ph. D. thesis, Massachusetts Institute of Technology, Boston, MA, USA (1995)
12. West, J., et al.: Comparison and evaluation of retrospective intermodality brain image registration techniques. J. Comput. Assist. Tomogr. 21(4), 554–566 (1997)
13. Zhang, J., Rangarajan, A.: Multimodality image registration using an extensible information metric and high dimensional histogramming. In: Christensen, G.E., Sonka, M. (eds.) IPMI 2005. LNCS, vol. 3565, pp. 725–737. Springer, Heidelberg (2005)

Simultaneous Brain Structures Segmentation Combining Shape and Pose Forces

Octavian Soldea[1], Trung Doan[2], Andrew Webb[3], Mark van Buchem[4],
Julien Milles[2], and Radu Jasinschi[1]

[1] Philips Research, Eindhoven, 5656AE, The Netherlands
octavian.soldea@philips.com
[2] Division of Image Processing, Department of Radiology, Leiden University
Medical Center, The Netherlands,
[3] CJ Gorter center for High Field MRI, Department of Radiology, Leiden University
Medical Center, The Netherlands,
[4] Department of Radiology, Leiden University Medical Center, The Netherlands

Abstract. This paper presents a new supervised learning based method for brain structure segmentation. We learn moment-based signatures of structures of interest and formulate the segmentation as a maximum a-posteriori estimation problem employing nonparametric multivariate kernel densities. For this problem, we propose a gradient flow solution. We have compared our method with state-of-the-art methods such as FSL-FIRST and Free-Surfer using volumetric 3T from IBSR. In addition, we have evaluated our algorithm on 7T MR data. We report comparative results of accuracy and significantly improved time-efficiency.

1 Introduction

The segmentation of brain structures in MR data, such as the hippocampus, putamen, and thalamus, is a challenge. For example, the hippocampus is a small structure that exhibits lack of contrast, whose shape changes in time according to how its various sub-structures manifest different atrophy rates which are correlated with the different stages of the evolution of Alzheimer's disease (AD) .

In the last ten years there has been an increase in the number of publications on the automatic segmentation of brain structures, and in particular, the hippocampus. In [1] a probabilistic method was shown, for which a posterior density is given by the product of an imaging model or data term probability and a prior term. The prior term is given by a mesh model whose structure is learned from a reference set. The parameter estimation is realized by the use of a generalized expectation-maximization method. In [2], the authors compare the performance of different (affine) registration methods aligning test and reference brains. They also compare the automatic hippocampus segmentation with that of manual segmentation.

The method proposed in this paper is based on active contours [3]. This approach has two main aspects. First, it combines the Chan-Vese [3] method, which extends the Mumford-Shah segmentation model to level sets, by adding

T. Liu et al. (Eds.): MBIA 2011, LNCS 7012, pp. 143–151, 2011.

to their data term a non-parametric prior shape term based on image moments. This is formulated as a probabilistic model, for which the estimated contours are computed based on the maximum a posteriori (MAP) of the posterior density. The prior density function is given by a set of (Gaussian) kernels which are a function of the difference between image moments computed for shape training sets and the ones for the testing set. Second, the segmentation of structures of interest is realized by taking into account their shape and pose inter-relationships in the context of multi-structure based methods. The pose, that is, location, size, and spatial orientation, which models the tight spatial interdependence of the brain structures, plays an important role in this multi-structure dependence [4]. Novel aspects in our method are:

1. The use of joint segmentation employing multi-structure shape and pose information in one unique and uniform mathematical framework, which is scalable at arbitrary resolutions,
2. A prior density that depends on the set of image moments only,
3. Registration is implicit to our segmentation method, a fact that has a strong effect on augmenting speed. Note that [5] cannot benefit from implicit registration due to the coupled shape forces model.
4. Most of the computational time in the segmentation process is used with the process of registration. To the best of our knowledge, this is the first method that uses implicit registration, and this does substantially reduce the computational time. We use moments in a different way than other contributions (see for example [6] and [7]).

In Section 2 we describe the theory and implementation of the proposed shape and pose prior based segmentation method. In Section 3 we present the experimental results, and in Section 4 we draw a conclusion.

2   Segmentation Based on Shape and Pose Priors

2.1   Overview of the Segmentation Algorithm

Given a test image, we initialize a set of candidate segmenting contours $C_{t=0}$ (we use t for indexing iterations, however, we avoid using it whenever it is not necessary). These contours (surfaces) are deformed by a linear combination of the Chan-Vese data term and the coupled shape and the relative pose prior forces in an iterative process. Note that while segmentation methods usually depend heavily on registration, here we use symbolic encoding of the pose. While the pose of structures of interest is described by moments based signatures, the natural outcome is a high increase in the computation speed. We describe the various steps in the segmentation algorithm in the flow diagram shown in Fig. 1 and Algorithm 1.

We align structures of interest employing pose. For example, the global orientation is given by that of the eigenvectors of the inertia matrix. Note that this moments based implementation of pose allows us to register an object to the absolute axes of coordinates. We call canonical the alignment defined by the mass center and inertia axes.

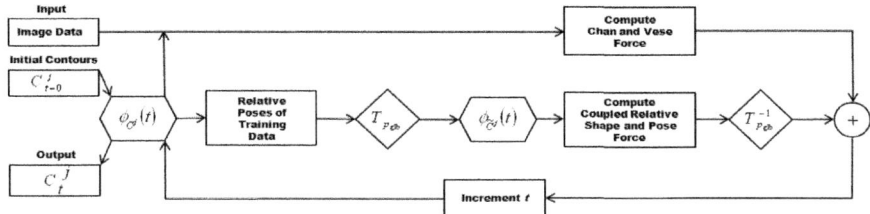

Fig. 1. Segmentation flow diagram. In each step, two forces are evaluated: the Chan-Vese and the coupled shape and relative pose components (see Section 2.3). T represents registration transformations.

Algorithm 1. Multi-Structure Segmentation Algorithm in Fig. 1

Input:
$t := 0$; $\mathbf{C}_{t=0}$; a training set of ensembles of structures $\tilde{C}_i$, where $i = \{1, \ldots, N\}$, and $\tilde{C}_i = \{\tilde{C}_i^1, \ldots, \tilde{C}_i^m\}$;
Δ_t; ε – a threshold for steady state
Output:
$\mathbf{C}_t$ a set of segmenting contours

  repeat
    for all j={1,\ldots,m}, (i.e. for each structure of interest) **do**
      1. Compute the data term of the Chan and Vese force, i.e. $\frac{\partial \phi_{CV}}{\partial t}$, for structure j of course, see also [3]
      2. Compute shape and relative pose according to Equation (9) :

$$\frac{\partial \phi_{\tilde{C}j}}{\partial t} := \frac{\sum\limits_{i=1}^{N} \prod\limits_{l=1}^{m} k_i^l \, MPF\,(j, i)\, \delta_\epsilon \left(\phi_{\tilde{C}j} \right)}{\sigma_j{}^2 \, P\left(\tilde{C} \right) \cdot N}$$

      3. Update the signed distance functions of each structure $\phi_{t+1} := \phi_t + \left(\frac{\partial \phi_{CV}}{\partial t} + \frac{\partial \phi_{\tilde{C}j}}{\partial t} \right) \cdot \Delta_t$

    end for
  until steady state is achieved, i.e. $d\left(\phi_t, \phi_{t+1} \right) < \varepsilon$, for all $j \in \{1, \ldots, m\}$

2.2   Probabilistic Formulation

Consider a set $\mathbf{C}$ of contours $\{C^1, ..., C^m\}$ that describe the boundaries, that is, surfaces, of m different brain structures for a given subject. These contours evolve according to the optimization process that minimizes a cost function or, equivalently, that maximize a probability density function. We have a set of N subjects, and therefore $\{\mathbf{C}_1, ..., \mathbf{C}_N\}$ contours; these define our training set. The set $\widetilde{\mathbf{C}}$ describes the contour set $\mathbf{C}$ augmented with pose information.

In our model we jointly represent the relative shape and pose. We do this by describing the contour information in terms of image moments, that is,

$$\widetilde{\mathbf{C}} = \left(p_{int}^1, ..., p_{int}^m \right), \tag{1}$$

where p_{int}^i represents the relative shape and pose information of each structure among these m structures. The parameters p_{int}^i are defined in terms of image moments.

We formulate the contour estimation as a MAP problem. The estimated contour set $\widehat{C}$ maximizes the posterior probability $P\left(\mathbf{C}|data\right) = \frac{P(data|\mathbf{C}) \times P(\mathbf{C}))}{P(data)}$, where we used Bayes' theorem. Since the (relative) inter-structure pose is independent of the global positioning of the brain, we assume that $P\left(\widetilde{\mathbf{C}}\right) = P\left(\mathbf{C}\right)$.

2.3   Coupled Shape and Pose Priors for Multi-structure Objects

We discuss here the expression for the prior contour term $\widetilde{\mathbf{C}}$. We define the joint kernel density estimate of m shapes as

$$P\left(\widetilde{\mathbf{C}}\right) = \frac{1}{N} \sum_{i=1}^{N} \prod_{j=1}^{m} k\left(d\left(\phi_{\widetilde{C}^j}, \phi_{\widetilde{C}_i^j}\right), \sigma_j\right), \tag{2}$$

where N is the number of training subjects and $k(., \sigma_j)$ is a Gaussian kernel with standard deviation σ_j. We use the index i to iterate through the training set. Similarly, we use j to iterate through the set of structures. The product in Equation (2) represents the coupling among structures.

In Equation (2), $\phi_{\widetilde{C}^j}$ is the test set signed distance function (SDF) of the jth structure, which is aligned to the training set, and $\phi_{\widetilde{C}_i^j}$ is the SDF of the ith training shape of the jth object.

In Equation (2), we use the distance metric:

$$d\left(\phi_1, \phi_2\right) = \sqrt{\sum_{r+s+t \leq L} w_{r,s,t} \left(m_{r,s,t}\left(\phi_1\right) - m_{r,s,t}\left(\phi_2\right)\right)^2}, \tag{3}$$

where $w_{r,s,t}$ are weights. In this context, in Section 2.4, we define for each SDF ϕ a sequence of moments $m_{r,s,t}\left(\phi\right)$, such that $r+s+t \leq L$, where L is a predefined constant.

Equation (2) is designed such that training shapes that are closer to $\widetilde{\mathbf{C}}$ contribute with higher weights. Furthermore, the products $\prod_{j=1}^{m} k\left(d\left(\phi_{\widetilde{C}^j}, \phi_{\widetilde{C}_i^j}\right), \sigma_j\right)$ exhibit coupling between the m individual structures to be segmented. This implies, for example, that a training sample (composed of curves for m structures) for which the k-th structure (where $k \in \{1 \ldots m\}$) is close to $\widetilde{\mathbf{C}}_k$ has relatively higher weights for the evolution of the other structures as well.

2.4   Moments and the Computation of the Shape and Pose

We compute the three-dimensional moment of order $r+s+t$, using the formula $m_{r,s,t} = \int_{\Omega} x^r y^s z^t f\left(x, y, z\right) dxdydz$, where r, s, t are integers and Ω is the volume of the structure. In particular, given the embedding function $\phi\left(x, y, z\right)$ of the object shape, where ϕ is a SDF, we define $f\left(x, y, z\right) = H\left(-\phi\left(x, y, z\right)\right)$; and $m_{r,s,t} = \int_{\Omega} x^r y^s z^t H\left(-\phi\left(x, y, z\right)\right) dxdydz$, where $H(\cdot)$ is the Heaviside function.

We now discuss the computation of the relative shape and pose variables in Equation (2) through moments. The relative shape and pose of the jth structure is given by:

$$p_{int}^j = \left[m_{0,0,0}^j, m_{1,0,0}^j, m_{0,1,0}^j, m_{0,0,1}^j, \cdots, m_{L,0,0}^j, m_{L-1,1,0}^j, \cdots, m_{0,0,L}^j\right]. \tag{4}$$

The distance in Equation (3) satisfies $d\left(\phi_{\widetilde{C}^j}, \phi_{\widetilde{C}^j_i}\right) = d\left(p^j_{int}, p^{ji}_{int}\right)$, so that Equation (2) becomes:

$$P(\widetilde{C}) = \frac{1}{N} \sum_{i=1}^{N} \prod_{j=1}^{m} k\left(d\left(p^j_{int}, p^{ji}_{int}\right), \sigma_j\right). \tag{5}$$

p^{ji}_{int} is the relative shape and pose of the jth structure of the ith training subject, whereas p^j_{int} is the relative shape and pose of the jth structure in the candidate (segmenting) ensemble of contours. We implement p^{ji}_{int} similarly to p^j_{int} in Equation (4). In both of the cases, we compute the moments of the jth structure of interest using the axis of the moments of inertia as the global coordinate system of reference. This implementation of pose represents implicit (or symbolic) registration. For estimation of σ_j we follow the method described in Section III of [5].

The Gaussian kernel functions in Equation (5) $\left(k^j_i \overset{\Delta}{=} k\left(d\left(p^j_{int}, p^{ji}_{int}\right), \sigma_j\right)\right)$ can be expressed as:

$$k^j_i = \frac{1}{\sqrt{2\pi\sigma_j{}^2}} \exp\left\{-\frac{1}{2\sigma_j{}^2}\left[\sum_{r+s+t \leq L} w^j_{r,s,t}\left(m^j_{r,s,t} - m^{ji}_{r,s,t}\right)^2\right]\right\}, \tag{6}$$

where $w^j_{r,s,t}$ are weights. We consider weights that sum up to one. Here, $m^j_{r,s,t}$ and $m^{ji}_{r,s,t}$ denote the moments of $\widetilde{C}^j$ and $\widetilde{C}^j_i$, respectively.

2.5   Gradient Flow of the Coupled Shape and Pose Prior

In this section, we define a gradient flow for the joint shape and pose prior in Equation (5). Given that $\log P\left(\widetilde{C}\right) = \log\left[\frac{1}{N}\sum_{i=1}^{N}\prod_{j=1}^{m} k^j_i\right]$, it can be shown that, for the kernel-based density in (2),

$$\frac{\partial}{\partial t}\log P\left(\widetilde{C}\right) = \frac{1}{N}\frac{\sum_{i=1}^{N}\left\{\sum_{j=1}^{m}\frac{\partial}{\partial t}k^j_i \prod_{l=1, l\neq j}^{m} k^l_i\right\}}{P\left(\widetilde{C}\right)}. \tag{7}$$

Using (6) and the fact that $m_{r,s,t} = \int_{\mathbb{R}^3} x^r y^s z^t H\left(-\phi\left(x,y,z\right)\right) dxdydz$ it can be shown that

$$\frac{\partial}{\partial t}k^j_i = \frac{k^j_i}{\sigma_j{}^2}\int_{\mathbb{R}^3}\sum_{m^j_{r,s,t}\in\mathcal{M}_L} w_{r,s,t}\, x^r y^s z^t\left[\left(m^j_{r,s,t} - m^{ji}_{r,s,t}\right)\delta_\epsilon\left(\phi_{\widetilde{C}^j}\right)\right]\frac{\partial\phi_{\widetilde{C}^j}}{\partial t}dxdydz. \tag{8}$$

Inserting (8) into (7), it can be shown that the solution $\widehat{C}$ to the MAP problem is obtained if

$$\frac{\partial\phi_{\widetilde{C}^j}}{\partial t} = \frac{\sum_{i=1}^{N}\prod_{l=1}^{m} k^l_i MPF\left(j,i\right)\delta_\epsilon\left(\phi_{\widetilde{C}^j}\right)}{\sigma_j{}^2 P\left(\widetilde{C}\right)\cdot N}, \tag{9}$$

is satisfied; $MPF(j,i) \equiv \sum_{r+s+t \leq L} w_{r,s,t}^{j} \, x^r y^s z^t \left(m_{r,s,t}^{j} - m_{r,s,t}^{ji} \right)$ for each $j \in \{1,\ldots,m\}$, and (x,y,z) denotes the spatial coordinates.

3   Experimental Results

We demonstrate our method on volumetric 3T and 7T MR data and perform a quantitative analysis of the accuracy of the segmentations in terms of Dice error rate (DC), relative volume difference ($RelVolDiff$) and the average surface distance ($AvgSrfDist$), as in [8]. We present experimental results on segmenting the left and right parts of the hippocampus (H), as well as the putamen (P), the caudate nucleus (CN), the globus pallidus (GlbPal), and the thalamus (Thlm). We compare the performance of our method on IBSR [9] (3T) data to state-of-the-art methods such as FSL-FIRST and Free-Surfer. Moreover, we have evaluated our algorithm on LeARN [10] (7T) data. We use ground truth shapes which are manually segmented by medical experts. We perform leave-one-out experiments and achieve steady state after fifty iterations, usually (we stop the processing at one hundred steps). In addition, we gradually increase the degree of moments from zero to higher orders; at each ten iterations we increase L (see also Equation (3)) by one. We also calibrate the weights to sum up to one and assign lower order moments higher weights. When segmenting multi-objects with $m = 2$, (see also Equation (1)), our method requires up to four minutes on a Core 2 Duo processor. We have implemented our scheme in C++ using ITK and VTK.

We performed several experiments on the IBSR [9] data set, in which there are 18 subjects: 14 male and 4 female. The ages of the subjects range from 7 to 71,

Table 1. Segmentation accuracy of Hippocampus on IBSR data in three experiments: Hippocampus (H) and Putamen (P); H and Caudate Nucleus (CN); and H, P, and CN

	DC	RelVolDiff	AvgSrfDist
Hippocampus and P	0.8165	0.3670	0.3756
Hippocampus and CN	0.8979	0.2042	0.2011
Hippocampus, CN, and P	0.9626	0.0747	0.0712

Table 2. Segmentation accuracy of left and right hippocampus on IBSR and LeARN data. The reported values are averages and standard deviations of absolute values measured for the analyzed subjects.

	Left Hippocampus			Right Hippocampus		
IBSR patients	DC	RelVolDiff	AvgSrfDist	DC	RelVolDiff	AvgSrfDist
Average	0.9338	0.1324	0.1463	0.9318	0.1365	0.1531
Standard Deviation	0.0557	0.1113	0.1339	0.0603	0.1207	0.1587

	Left Hippocampus			Right Hippocampus		
7T patients	DC	RelVolDiff	AvgSrfDist	DC	RelVolDiff	AvgSrfDist
Average	0.7969	0.2664	0.2581	0.9251	0.1497	0.1177
Standard Deviation	0.0395	0.0286	0.0200	0.0337	0.0675	0.0725

Table 3. A comparison of the proposed method with state-of-the-art methods such as FSL-FIRST and Free-Surfer. Each line labeled with Proposed Method means a leave-one-out experiment on IBSR data, where the completed squares represent a coupling among the marked structures.

Method / DC of Structure	CN	P	Thlm	GlbPal	AccN	H
Proposed Method	0.9650	0.9803		0.8607		0.9536
Proposed Method				0.7860		0.9524
Free Surfer	0.8208	0.8255	0.8550	0.7826	0.5850	0.7703
FSL-FIRST	0.8164	0.8868	0.8179	0.6600	0.5688	0.7609

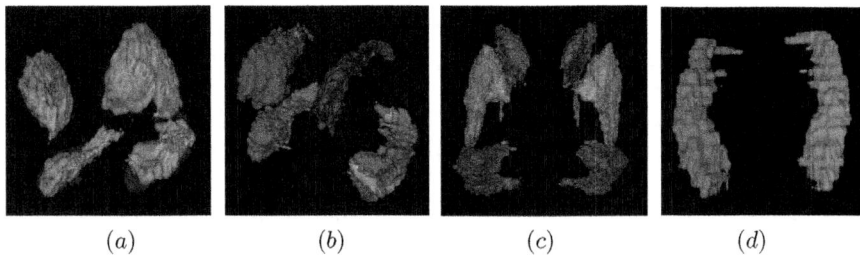

(a)   *(b)*   *(c)*   *(d)*

Fig. 2. Segmentation results on IBSR data superimposed to ground truth (yellow). Images $(a), (b)$, and (c) represent couplings of H with CN, H with P, and H with CN and P, respectively. In image (d), the red and blue hippocampus parts appear as gray and orange due to being superimposed to the ground truth in yellow.

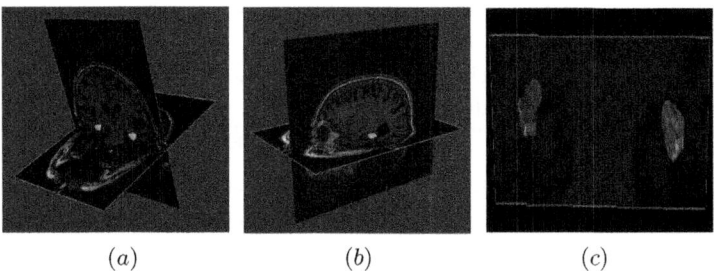

(a)   *(b)*   *(c)*

Fig. 3. Segmentation in 7T MR data using the color coding in Fig. 2 (d). Images (a) and (b) illustrate ground truth of the hippocampus body. Image (c) shows an automatic segmentation result of left and right parts of hippocampus body.

the resolution is 256x256x128, and the spacing is 0.94x0.94x1.5 mm. In the first three experiments, we consider the couplings: H with P, H with CN, and H with CN and P. We report results of accuracy of segmentation in Table 1 and illustrate examples in Figures 2 $(a), (b)$, and (c), respectively. These experiments show that more coupling provides better accuracy, see the DC column. In a fourth experiment, we focus on left and right hippocampus segmentation. We report results of accuracy of segmentation in Table 2 and illustrate an example in

Fig. 2 (d). In addition we have performed a set of experiments in which we group CN, P, GlbPal, and H and compared the results with state-of-the-art methods such as FSL-FIRST and Free-Surfer. We show these results in Table 3 and report improved accuracy as compared to FSL and Free-Surfer as well as faster computation times.

We have also performed a quantitative analysis on 7T T1 MR images, courtesy of Leiden University Medical Center. We have selected a cohort of nine images with a resolution of 256x256x60 and spacing of 0.98x0.98x3 mm. While in IBSR, we have a spacing of 1.5 mm in the coronary direction, here, the 3mm value is in the axial orientation. We report results of accuracy of segmentation of the hippocampus body in Table 2 and illustrate ground truth and an example in Fig. 3. While the training set is much more restricted as compared to the experiments on IBSR we report comparable accuracy and similar time requirements.

4 Conclusion

We have presented a multi-modal density learning-based statistical approach for segmentation of multiple basal ganglia structures and the hippocampus. Our main contributions are: (i) design of new prior density terms, (ii) coupled densities of multiple structures, (iii) use of implicit registration, which has a strong effect on augmenting speed, and (iv) a unique platform for the joint shape and pose modeling. We have presented experimental results on 3T and 7T MR data and compared our approach to current state-of-the-art methods, such as FSL and Free-Surfer. We report significant improvements of both accuracy and time-efficiency as compared to state-of-the-art approaches. The method allows for an elegant fusion between different MR contrasts. For future investigation, we intend to generalize our method by employing statistical information of image intensities while preserving its time-efficiency.

Acknowledgment. This research was performed within the framework of CTMM, the Center for Translational Molecular Medicine [10], project LeARN (grant 02N-101).

References

1. Leemput, K.V., Bakkour, A., Benner, T., Wiggins, G., Wald, L.L., Augustinack, J., Dickerson, B.C., Golland, P., Fischl, B.: Automated segmentation of hippocampal subfields from ultra-high resolution in vivo mri. HIPPOCAMPUS 19, 549–557 (2009)
2. Carmichael, O., Aizenstein, H.A., Davis, S., Becker, J., Thompson, P., Meltzer, C., Liu, Y.: Atlas-based hippocampus segmentation in alzheimer's disease and mild cognitive impairment. NeuroImage 27, 979–990 (2005)
3. Chan, T.F., Vese, L.A.: Active contours without edges. IEEE Transactions on Image Processing 10, 266–277 (2001)

4. Styner, M., Gorczowski, K., Fletcher, T., Jeong, J.Y., Pizer, S.M., Gerig, G.: Statistics of pose and shape in multi-object complexes using principal geodesic analysis. In: Yang, G.-Z., Jiang, T.-Z., Shen, D., Gu, L., Yang, J. (eds.) MIAR 2006. LNCS, vol. 4091, pp. 1–8. Springer, Heidelberg (2006)
5. Uzunbaş, M.G., Soldea, O., Ünay, D., Çetin, M., Ünal, G., Erçil, A., Ekin, A.: Coupled non-parametric shape and moment-based inter-shape pose priors for multiple basal ganglia structure segmentation. IEEE Transactions on Medical Imaging 29(12), 1959–1978 (2010)
6. Foulonneau, A., Charbonnier, P., Heitz, F.: Affine-invariant geometric shape priors for region-based active contours. IEEE Transactions on Pattern Analysis and Machine Intelligence 28(8), 1352–1357 (2006)
7. Huang, F., Su, J.: Moment-based shape priors for geometric active contours. In: The 18th IEEE International Conference on Pattern Recognition, vol. 2, pp. 56–59 (2006)
8. Heimann, T., Heimann, T., Styner, M.: Evaluation measures, http://mbi.dkfz-heidelberg.de/grand-challenge2007/sites/eval.htm
9. IBSR: Internet Brain Segmentation Repository, www.cma.mgh.harvard.edu/ibsr/
10. CTMM: Center for translational molecular medicine, www.ctmm.nl

Improved Tissue Segmentation by Including an MR Acquisition Model

Dirk H.J. Poot[1], Marleen de Bruijne[1,2], Meike W. Vernooij[4],
M. Arfan Ikram[1,4], and Wiro J. Niessen[1,3]

[1] BIGR, Erasmus Medical Center, Rotterdam, The Netherlands
[2] Department of Computer Science, University of Copenhagen, Denmark
[3] Delft University of Technology, Delft, The Netherlands
[4] Department of Epidemiology & Department of Radiology, Erasmus MC, Rotterdam

Abstract. This paper presents a new MR tissue segmentation method. In contrast to most previous methods the image formation model includes the point spread function of the image acquisition. This allows optimal combination of images acquired with different contrast weighting, resolutions, and orientations. The proposed method computes the regularized maximum likelihood partial volume segmentation from the images. The quality the resulting segmentation is studied with a simulation experiment and by testing the reproducibility of the segmentation on repeated brain MRI scans. Our results demonstrate improved segmentation quality, especially at tissue edges.

Keywords: Tissue segmentation, multi modal imaging, point spread function.

1 Introduction

Tissue segmentation is an important task for quantitative medical image analysis. Previously published approaches perform tissue segmentation on (resampled) voxel intensities of typically one [1,2,3,4,5,6] or sometimes multiple images with different contrast weighting directly [7,8]. However, when the resolution or orientation of images with different contrast weighting differs, segmenting based on the resampled voxel intensities leads to inconsistencies in the information, especially at tissue borders and small scale structures that might not be resolved by all images. By taking the point spread function (PSF) of the individual acquisitions into account, these inconsistencies can be avoided, thereby improving the segmentation result.

Several methods that estimate partial volume (PV) segmentations have been proposed [4,7,6]. These PV segmentation methods aim to improve segmentation at tissue borders. However, except for [6] where a smoothed segmentation is sought, these methods assume voxels to integrate the signal emitted inside a box in space. While integrating over a box might be appropriate for some imaging systems, it is only a rough approximation for the MR imaging process in which explicitly a part of k-space is acquired. Additionally, these methods do

T. Liu et al. (Eds.): MBIA 2011, LNCS 7012, pp. 152–159, 2011.

not account for intrinsic resolution differences of the multi modal images used for classification.

In this paper, a PV tissue segmentation is proposed that in addition to the bias field [1, 3, 9] also accounts for the PSF and resolution differences of each of the MR images. This new method is validated by simulation experiments and the reproducibility is tested on repeated acquisitions of brain MR images.

2   Methods

2.1   Model of the Object

For the tissue segmentation we assume that the object $O(x)$ consists of a small number of m tissues. At each location, the element $k \in [1 \ldots m]$ of $O(x)$, denoted by $O_k(x)$, specifies the fraction of tissue present at location x that is of class k. Although at each location only one tissue is present, this formulation allows the reconstruction from images with a finite resolution. Since it is assumed that all tissues in the region of interest are modeled, the fractional contributions should sum to one, $\sum_k O_k(x) = 1$. The aim of the tissue segmentation is estimation of $O(x)$ from a set of MR images of an object.

The model of the magnitude of the signal received from each point of the object when acquiring the j-th image is given by by:

$$M_j(x) = \sum_k O_k(x) V_{k,j} B_j(x; b_j), \tag{1}$$

where $V_{k,j}$ is the (mean) intensity of the tissue types in MR image $j \in [1 \ldots N]$ and $B_j(x; b_j)$ is the bias field which is parametrized by b_j ($n_{p_j} \times 1$). The bias-field captures sensitivity inhomogeneities of the receive coils as well as (small) transmit inhomogeneities. If the latter distortions are large, as might happen in high field MRI, relative constrasts might change. This is currently not modelled.

2.2   Model of the MRI Acquisition

MR images of the brain are most commonly acquired with multi-slice imaging methods. For each slice of a multi-slice MR image, the MR acquisition records a part of the k-space. The image of a slice is then reconstructed by the discrete Fourier transform. These two steps are equivalent to convolving the object with the 3D PSF, followed by sampling at each of the grid nodes of the MR image. Thus a model of the MR image acquisition is given by

$$S_j(y) = \int M_j(x) w(T_j(x; t_j) - y) dx + e_j(y) \tag{2}$$

$$\approx \sum_q M_j(x_q) w(T_j(x_q; t_j) - y) + e_j(y), \tag{3}$$

where for each different contrast encoding j, M_j ($n_M \times 1$) is a vector containing the intensities of the continuous M_j at the 3D grid points x_q, $q \in \{1, \ldots, n_{M_j}\}$, where x_q is a coordinate in object space. Furthermore, S_j $(n_{S_j} \times 1)$ is a vector containing the samples of the jth contrast encoded MR image S_j at the grid nodes y_l, $l \in \{1, \dots, n_{S_j}\}$, where y_l is a coordinate in the space of the jth MR image. The measurement noise e_j $(n_{S_j} \times 1)$ is assumed to be $\sim \mathcal{N}(0, I\sigma_j^2)$, i.e. independent, normally distributed with zero mean and standard deviation σ_j. This is an acceptable assumption as the signal magnitude of the MR images for all (interesting) tissue types is $> 3\sigma_j$. The coordinate transformation T_j links x and y and is parametrized by t_j $(n_{t_j} \times 1)$ to allow for potential subject movement between the different acquisitions. Finally, w is the PSF, which is (implicitly) defined by the MR image acquisition grid and depends on the slice orientation. For multi slice acquisition methods that sample a rectangular part of the k-space with sufficient density, this sampling function can be split into three functions that are applied in orthogonal directions that are aligned with the MR- image coordinates, $w(y) = \prod_{i=1}^{3} w_i(y_i)$. Lets assume, without loss of generality, that the coordinates y_i are ordered 1, 2 and 3 for read encoding, phase encoding, and slice encoding, respectively. Then, due to the rectangular part of k-space that is sampled, w_1 and w_2 are Dirichlet, or periodic sinc, functions, possibly scaled to account for zero filling in k-space. For multi-slice MR images, w_3 depends on the slice selection of the acquisition method. Slice selection is often performed by either a (windowed) sinc or a Gaussian shaped RF pulse, so the sampling in the slice direction w_3 can be modeled by a (smoothed) box or Gaussian function, respectively. In our experiments, with windowed sinc slice excitation, w_3 was modeled with a smoothed box function :

$$
w_3(y) = \begin{cases} 1 & |y| \leq \frac{1}{3} \\ \frac{1}{2} - \frac{1}{2}\sin\left(3\pi(|y| - \frac{1}{2})\right) & \frac{1}{3} < |y| < \frac{2}{3} \\ 0 & \frac{2}{3} \leq |y| \end{cases} \tag{4}
$$

Alternatively, the excitation profile w_3 can be measured by a dedicated acquisition. Eq. (3) is efficiently evaluated by the method described in [10].

2.3   Likelihood Function

The likelihood function of the MR images can be used to quantify the quality of the fit between segmentation and the images. Since the noise is assumed to be Gaussian distributed and independent, the log likelihood function is given by:

$$
L(O, \Theta|S) = \sum_{j,l} \frac{-1}{2\sigma_j^2} \left(\sum_q w(T_j(x_q; t_j) - y_l) \sum_k O(x_q, k) V_{k,j} B_j(x_q; b_j) - S_j(y_l) \right)^2,
$$

$$\tag{5}$$

where $\Theta = [V_{j,k} \; b_j^T \; t_j^T \; (\forall j, k)]^T$. Since we are only interested in locations of maxima of L, the constant offset term $\frac{-1}{2}\sum_j N_{S_j} \ln\left(2\pi\sigma_j^2\right)$ is ignored in Eq. (5).

2.4   Regularization of the Solution

Since the number of variables might exceed the number of measurements, the solution might be under determined or badly conditioned. Therefore, a regularization is applied. In a Bayesian framework the regularization is the prior distribution for the segmented objectin the space of all possible segmentations. For tissue segmentation neighboring voxels are likely to be of the same class and a voxel often contains one tissue class, which is realized by:

$$R(\boldsymbol{O}) = \sum_{q,q',k} O_k(\boldsymbol{x}_q) O_k(\boldsymbol{x}_{q'}) F(\boldsymbol{x}_q - \boldsymbol{x}_{q'}), \tag{6}$$

where $R(\boldsymbol{O})$ is the logarithm of the un-normalized prior distribution and $F(\boldsymbol{x}_q - \boldsymbol{x}_{q'})$ specifies the contribution to the likelihood when two voxels $\boldsymbol{x}_q$ and $\boldsymbol{x}_{q'}$ both have a fraction of tissue k. By selecting an appropriate positive value for $F(\boldsymbol{0})$, the prior for a single tissue type per voxel is specified, while positive values for F when $\boldsymbol{x}_q$ is a neighbor of $\boldsymbol{x}_{q'}$ specify the likelihood that neighboring voxels contain the same tissue type. The scaling factors F explicitly do not depend on k nor on the actual position $\boldsymbol{x}_q$ to make sure that each tissue is treated equally and spatially independent, thus a low amount of prior knowledge is included in the segmentation method. In our implementation F was a filter containing a weighted sum of Gaussian blurring, voxel based Laplacian, and a constant added to $F(0)$. The weighting parameters, constant, and the width of the Gaussian kernel were optimized by minimizing the mean square error (MSE) in the simulation experiment described in Section 3.

2.5   Optimization

The tissue classification is the solution of a constrained maximization problem:

$$\hat{\boldsymbol{O}}, \hat{\boldsymbol{\Theta}} = \arg \max_{\substack{\boldsymbol{O}, \boldsymbol{\Theta} \\ \boldsymbol{O} \geq 0 \\ \sum_k O(\boldsymbol{x}_q, k) = 1}} L(\boldsymbol{O}, \boldsymbol{\Theta} | \boldsymbol{S}) + R(\boldsymbol{O}). \tag{7}$$

Solving the optimization problem Eq. (7) is not easy since the number of parameters is large and the combined problem of optimizing $\boldsymbol{O}$ and $\boldsymbol{\Theta}$ is non-linear. Therefore, the following optimization procedure was developed:

1. An initial hard segmentation $\boldsymbol{O}$ is created by resampling each MR image to the grid $\boldsymbol{x}_q$ and assigning each voxel to the tissue type whose class center was closest. The distance measure was weighted by the noise level in each image.
2. With this initial segmentation, Eq. (7) is locally optimized with respect to $\boldsymbol{\Theta}$. The optimization is performed in MATLAB with the non linear least squares optimization routine lsqnonlin and a custom routine that computes the terms in Eq. (5) before squaring, as well as their derivative.
3. Eq. (7) is optimized with respect to $\boldsymbol{O}$, starting from the initial segmentation and $\boldsymbol{\Theta}$ estimated in the step 2. In this case $L + R$ reduces to the quadratic form $\boldsymbol{O}^T \boldsymbol{A} \boldsymbol{O} + \boldsymbol{B}^T \boldsymbol{O} + C$, with $\boldsymbol{A}$ $(Nn_M \times Nn_M)$, $\boldsymbol{B}$ $(Nn_M \times 1)$, and C scalar. However, since A is not necessarily negative definite it is impossible to guarantee that the global maximum is found. For efficient handling

of the structured constraints a custom optimization routine, based on [11] and active set optimization was developed. The method alternated between optimizing a constrained sub problem with the conjugated gradient method followed by an update of the set of constraints that are enforced.

3   Experiments and Results

This section evaluates the proposed method with a simulation experiment and by segmenting the MR images of subjects from a population study [12].

3.1   Phantom Experiment

For this experiment a 3D phantom object was constructed, see Fig. 1(a). In this object some sharp features are present, but most 'tissue' edges are smooth curves. In this respect this artificial object is quite representative for many biological tissue configurations. Each of the 6 classes is assigned a random color in each of the three differently oriented MR images, representing images with different contrast weightings. See Fig. 1(b) for the resampled simulated images to which a low amount of noise was added. See Fig. 1(c) for the result of step 1, which is a segmentation of Fig. 1(b). When the class labels are optimized with Eq. (7), the segmentation quality is improved, as can be seen in Fig. 1(d). Fig. 1(e) shows that the nearest mean classification has many more classification errors at tissue borders than the proposed method, which is due to the interpolation and Gibbs ringing in the MR images. Fig. 1(f) shows that only occasionally PV voxels are selected in this simulation in which the ground truth is discrete. Furthermore, if a wrong class has the maximum PV, its PV typically is relatively small.

3.2   Brain MR Images

For in vivo brain measurements the ground truth segmentation is not known. Therefore, the reproducibility of the new segmentation method is evaluated on images of 7 persons that have been scanned twice with approximately 7 days between the scans. From the acquired MR images, three multi slice images were selected for the tissue segmentation task: A T1 weighted image with an intrinsic in-plane resolution (Acquisition matrix) of 416 x 256 voxels and 96 slices, voxel size 1.2 mm x 2.0 mm x 2.0 mm. A Fast spin echo (FSE) image with the same resolution and voxel size, but with a field of view (FOV) that was rotated by approximately 5 degrees; A Fluid Attenuated Inversion Recovery (FLAIR) image with an in-plane resolution of 320 x 224 and 64 slices, voxel dimensions 1.6 mm x 2.3 mm x 2 mm. The orientation of the FOV was equal to the FSE image. In the segmentation 5 tissue classes were used: cerebrospinal fluid (CSF), gray matter (GM), white matter (WM), white matter lesion (WML) and blood vessel (BV). The WML/GM intensity was kept at 1 for the T1 and FSE image, and 1.6 for the FLAIR image. The intensity of WML should be constrained as it is not necessarily present in the images. From the images the PV segmentation is

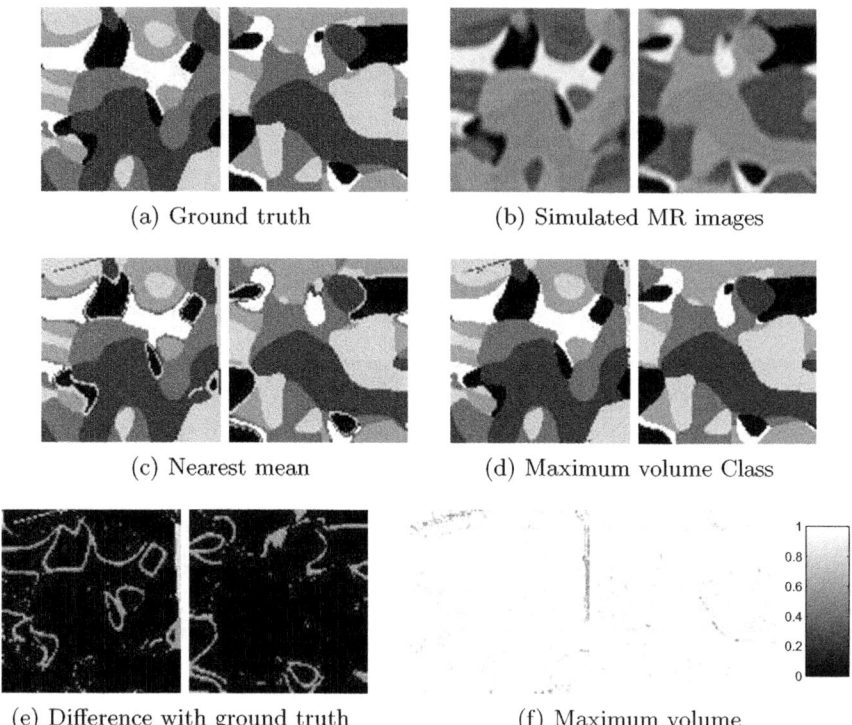

(a) Ground truth   (b) Simulated MR images

(c) Nearest mean   (d) Maximum volume Class

(e) Difference with ground truth   (f) Maximum volume

Fig. 1. Simulated 3D object classification experiment. Each subfigure displays identical orthogonal planes through the center. (a) shows the ground truth tissue classes. (b) shows the resampled simulated MR images, each assigned to a different color channel (RGB). (c) shows the nearest mean class (NM). (d) shows the maximum PV class (mPV). (e) shows the voxels in which NM (green) and mPV (red) differ from the ground truth class. (f) shows the maximum PV in each voxel.

computed on a grid aligned with the T1 image, but with voxel size of 0.8mm x 0.8 mm x 0.8mm and dimensions large enough to cover the brain and skull.

Fig. 2 shows the results of a random subject. The segmentation obtained by a state of the art automatically trained brain tissue segmentation method [8] is shown as reference. In order to display the same anatomical locations in Fig. 2, the two scans are registered (affine) and all segmentations are transformed to the mean space. One of the differences of the proposed method w.r.t. the other methods is the removal of GM above and below the ventricles, which most likely is anatomically correct. This difference in classification is due to incorporation of the PSF in the PV segmentation. The edge effect which causes the nearest mean, and the method of [8] to classify these voxels as GM is the same as in the simulation study described in the subsection 3.1. For each subject, the relative mean difference in segmentation, $r_k = \frac{\sum_{q \in \Omega} |O_k^1(\boldsymbol{x}_q) - O_k^2(\boldsymbol{x}_q)|}{\sum_{q \in \Omega} O_k^1(\boldsymbol{x}_q) + O_k^2(\boldsymbol{x}_q)}$, between the registered segmentations of the first (O_k^1) and second (O_k^2) time points was

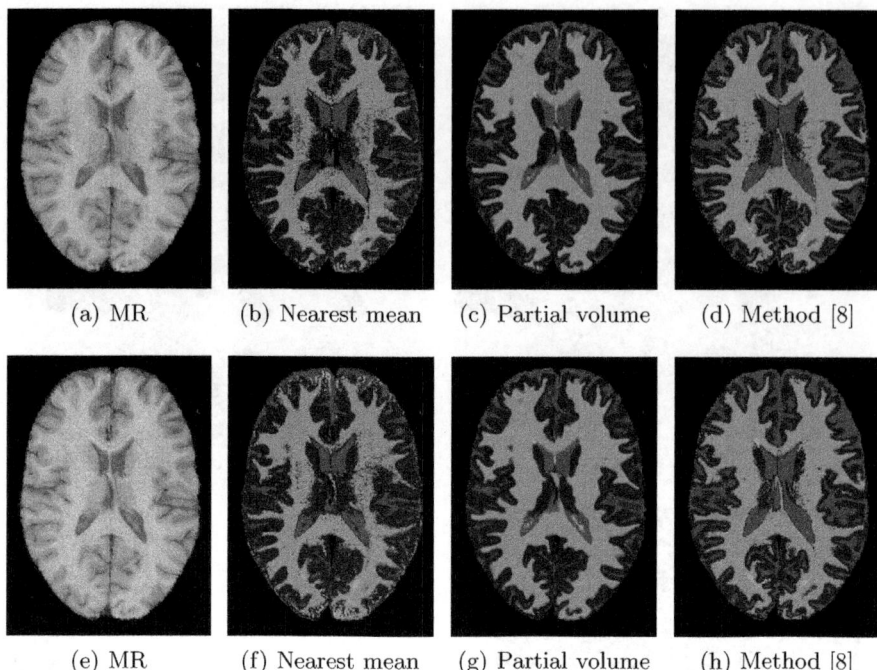

(a) MR   (b) Nearest mean   (c) Partial volume   (d) Method [8]

(e) MR   (f) Nearest mean   (g) Partial volume   (h) Method [8]

Fig. 2. This figure shows an axial slice of the biasfield corrected resampled MR images (R:FSE, G:T1, B:FLAIR) (a, e), the classification results of the reproducibility test with the nearest mean segmentation (b, f), the proposed PV segmentation (c, g), and the segmentation method proposed in [8] (d, h). The same slice of the first (a, b, c, d) and second dataset (e, f, g, h) is displayed. The CSF (red), Gray matter (blue), white matter (green), WML (cyan) and blood vessel (black) classes are displayed. A brain mask has been applied to remove erroneous classification outside the brain.

computed, within the brain mask Ω. The mean and standard deviation of r_k for the gray and white matter was for the proposed method: 0.073 ± 0.017, 0.063 ± 0.011 and for the method of [8]: 0.223 ± 0.017, 0.167 ± 0.011, respectively. This is indicative of a substantial improvement in reproducibility by the proposed method. However, this comparison might be biased as [8] does not estimate PV segmentations and does impose less spatial regularization, thus potentially being slightly more sensitive to residual registration errors.

4   Discussion and Conclusion

The results show a good quality segmentation of the simulated phantom. Specifically, by inclusion of the PSF of the acquisition within the segmentation procedure, the classification errors at the tissue borders of the nearest mean classifier are automatically removed. The experiment with real MR images also indicates improved and more reproducable segmentation when compared to the nearest mean classification and the segmentation method proposed in [8].

To conclude, we proposed a new method for tissue segmentation from multi modal images acquired with different orientations and resolutions. Compared to methods that perform a voxel based classification of resampled images, this method improves the segmentation by taking the point spread functions of the different images into account. Simulation experiments as well as segmentations of brain MR images demonstrated improvements in segmentation quality and reproducibility, compared to direct voxel intensity based segmentation methods. These improvements are especially located at tissue borders, where interpolation creates intensity values that might be classified erroneously.

References

1. Kapur, T., et al.: Segmentation of brain tissue from magnetic resonance images. Medical Image Analysis 1(2), 109–127 (1996)
2. Tasdizen, T., et al.: MRI tissue classification with neighborhood statistics: A nonparametric, entropy-minimizing approach. In: Duncan, J.S., Gerig, G. (eds.) MICCAI 2005. LNCS, vol. 3750, pp. 517–525. Springer, Heidelberg (2005)
3. Van Leemput, K., et al.: Automated model-based bias field correction of MR images of the brain. IEEE T. Med. Imaging 18(10), 885–896 (1999)
4. Van Leemput, K., et al.: A unifying framework for partial volume segmentation of brain MR images. IEEE T. Med. Imaging 22(1), 105–119 (2003)
5. Zhang, Y., et al.: Segmentation of brain MR images through a hidden markov random field model and the expectation-maximization algorithm. IEEE T. Med. Imaging 20(1), 45–57 (2001)
6. Pham, D.L., Prince, J.L.: Unsupervised partial volume estimation in single-channel image data. In: IEEE Workshop on Mathematical Methods in Biomedical Image Analysis, p. 170 (2000)
7. Pokric, M., et al.: Multi-dimensional medical image segmentation with partial voluming. In: Proc. MIUA, pp. 77–81 (2001)
8. Cocosco, C.A., et al.: A fully automatic and robust brain MRI tissue classification method. Medical Image Analysis 7(4), 513–527 (2003)
9. Wells, W.M., et al.: Adaptive segmentation of MRI data. IEEE T. Med. Imaging 15(4), 429–442 (1996)
10. Poot, D.H.J., et al.: General and efficient super-resolution method for multi-slice MRI. In: Jiang, T., Navab, N., Pluim, J.P.W., Viergever, M.A. (eds.) MICCAI 2010. LNCS, vol. 6361, pp. 615–622. Springer, Heidelberg (2010)
11. Byrd, R.H., et al.: A trust region method based on interior point techniques for nonlinear programming. Mathematical Programming 89(1), 149–185 (2000)
12. Hofman, A., et al.: The rotterdam study: 2010 objectives and design update. Eur. J. Epidemiol. 24(9), 553–572 (2009)

Author Index